DISCOVER A HEALTHY YOU

Your Life, My Guidance:
Inspiration, Reflection, and Action

DISCOVER A HEALTHY YOU

Your Life, My Guidance:
Inspiration, Reflection, and Action

Katie Tedder

Published by:

Katydid Fitness Publishing

Requests for permissions should be addressed to the author via email, katy.katydidfitness@gmail.com

ISBN: [978-1-7339907-0-7]

First Edition: April 20, 2019
Printed in the United States of America

About KatydidFitness.com

KatydidFitness.com is a resource dedicated to helping women navigate through their own health & fitness journey. You can find workout and nutrition books, as well as, exercise videos at all different levels of fitness.

I welcome you to enjoy and participate in my Facebook community: **www.Facebook.com/KatydidFitness**

Find other written works on Katie Tedder's author page on Amazon:

www.amazon.com/author/katietedder

This book is dedicated to all women who are on their own health journey; You are worthy. Never give up!

TABLE OF CONTENTS

ACKNOWLEDGEMENT

I've always been a girl who followed the path she thought she was supposed to take. God provided me with the gift of teaching, so I pursued that career. Little did I know, I was destined to discover so many aspects of teaching.

I started as an Elementary Education teacher. That's where I initially thought my identity would lie, but after becoming a stay at home mom, I explored Network Marketing teaching and leading a team of women. I am teaching my children at home to prepare them for school. My journey has led me to rediscover my love for fitness and am now personally training and coach ing women around the world. I love using my writing to help teach women about health & fitness.

With that said, I must thank some important people in my life:

I thank God for gifting me the talent of teaching, in order to help so many individuals. I will always think of myself as a teacher, before a writer, but the avenues in which I teach are many.

Thank you Will, for supporting me through this journey. You are my best friend and always want the best for me. Thank you for providing for our family, so I can pursue my dream.

To my parents, Sandra and Roy, thank you so much for always believing in me and encouraging me to always do my best and strive for more. You two are the reason I am as dedicated and determined as I am today. Your love and support means the world to me. And thanks dad for helping with this project.

I want to thank my sister Amy, for always being there for me. Sure, you loved giving me a hard time, as kids, but you helped prepare me for the real world of criticism and always stuck up for me when it mattered. I love you.

To My Friends, Thank you all so much for encouraging me and being my support system for so long. Having the support from close friends is priceless when trying to achieve goals. You all have been there for me through thick and thin and I am truly grateful.

To everyone who I've crossed paths with, thank you for being in my life, even for a brief moment. I am a true believer that God places people in our lives for a reason, so I know that everyone that I have and will encounter will have an impact on my life and journey.

PREFACE

I love journaling and devotional books. I love books that allow the reader to reflect on an issue or topic that applies to one's own life. I am a Certified Fitness and Nutrition Coach through the International Sports Sciences Association (ISSA), and I have found so many women that just don't know where to begin when it comes to their own health and fitness journey. They buy a pre-made plan and try it for a week or two and then go back to their own habits because their life is just too crazy and they can't keep up with it all. They haven't learned how to build a strong foundation for their health and fitness goals. They haven't learned how to form and sustain good habits.

No matter what age you are, I'm sure you have a to-do list a mile long. That's what women are great at, right? Another thing we are great at is giving our time to everyone else, EXCEPT OURSELVES! We put ourselves on the back burner while we cook, clean, go to work, help with homework, run kids from activity to activity, while doing loads of laundry, etc. Finding time to even sit down is a rarity. I get it. I have 3 kids of my own and a husband who works crazy hours. As much as we need to be flexible; I'm here to tell you that it IS POSSIBLE to still give yourself some time and work on your health. It IS POSSIBLE to become the woman you want to be amidst the crazy life you may have. It just takes organization and focus.

And that, my friend, is why I wrote this book. I will help you break down your busy schedule and help you figure out how and what to do in order to move in a healthy direction. This is NOT a transformation plan! This book is NOT a one size fits all, I'll tell you what to do, and it will magically work plan! With this book, I will give you the tools to figure out your own plan that works for YOU. I hope to use positivity, inspiration, and my experience in order to help you to look at your OWN life…did you hear that? No One Else's…and to reflect, write, and learn how to incorporate good habits that will help you discover a healthy YOU!

Chapter 1

YOUR WAY TO AN OVERALL HEALTHIER LIFESTYLE

"Accept responsibility for your life. Know that it is you who will get you where you want to go, no one else." -Les Brown

Take a deep breath. It's time to start your health and fitness journey. Nervousness may be setting in. Maybe you are feeling anxiety or doubt about the whole process. Hopefully you are also feeling some excitement as well! Whatever you are feeling right now, don't let it stop you from trying.

I am here to help you learn and apply three components (mindset, exercise, and nutrition) and walk this journey with you to help you be successful with your goals. Yes, it can feel scary. You may feel defeated before you even begin, because you feel that your goals are too far out of reach right now. You don't know how you will ever achieve them. It is okay to feel that way! You're not alone! I will help you put that all at ease. Mindset, Exercise, and Nutrition work together; however, if you work on any one of these

1

components, I truly believe that you will be on your way to a healthier lifestyle.

I have structured this book down into easy to read chapters to help you think about the components as they apply to your own life and how you can incorporate them properly to form better habits in your daily and weekly routine.

After each chapter, I will provide you with time to reflect on the topic as it speaks to your own life. I encourage you to think about how you can incorporate or start certain things on a small scale to eventually form good habits towards your health journey. It takes around 21 days to form a habit... good or bad. I will challenge you to incorporate small tasks for 21 days to help you form those good habits that will improve your health journey. When you complete the task you mark it off on the record sheet I provide you. I will also provide some examples as to what I mean, when I get to that portion in the book.

Please know that these tasks are not elaborate. They are all reasonable and possible to fit into a day if you think about it a little bit. That's why we're here right? To Discover a Healthy You! You know your life better than anyone. You are in charge! If you apply these components into your daily/weekly routine and they become a habit, over time you will discover the healthy you that you are looking for! Are you ready?!

Chapter 2

YOUR MINDSET

"A healthy outside starts from the inside."
-Robert Urich

The mind is a very powerful thing. Just one thought can make or ruin our day. Our mindset is our belief about ourselves and abilities. A person who has a negative mindset probably uses the words can't, shouldn't, never, no, impossible, don't. They may even say, "I WISH I could." These words seem harmless, but they destroy our image about ourselves and ultimately delay progress. "I can't do a push up." "Oh, I shouldn't sign up for this race, because it takes time away from my family." "I will never be able to lose this weight." "No, I don't have time." "Getting 30 minutes to myself is impossible." "Oh, I wish I could feel healthy enough to play on the floor with my kids/grandkids."

If you say or think any of these things (or anything like it) on a regular basis, then we need to work on your mindset. First off, you need to know that YOU CAN! YOU SHOULD! YOU WILL! IT IS POSSIBLE! YOU ARE CAPABLE! You may not see it now, but as we work through the strategies I lay out for you, you will find those little pockets of time that you never thought you had. You will find yourself celebrating your successes…no matter how big or small. You will start seeing yourself as a strong, confident woman, who is capable of anything if you just take those small steps and keep working towards your goals.

It's Time To Reflect! This is the time to be honest. Honesty about yourself is only going to help you figure out what you need to work so you can then make improvements.

What words do you find yourself saying about your image?

What words do you find yourself saying about your abilities?

What words do you find yourself saying about your time?

What words do you find yourself saying about your health?

What words do you find yourself saying about life in general?

Based on how you answered above, do you feel that you have a positive or negative mindset?

Now that you are aware of your mindset, let us dive into how you can incorporate a positive mindset into your daily routines.

If you already have a positive mindset, then you will want to make sure you are incorporating the ideas I present in the upcoming chapters into your routine. You don't want to slip into a negative mindset if something doesn't go your way. You want to be able to be flexible and positively adjust to whatever comes your way.

If you have a negative mindset, then these upcoming chapters are crucial for you to build a solid starting foundation in your overall health and fitness journey. I encourage you to really take the reflection time seriously and take the time you need to incorporate these ideas into your life until you have really created a positive habit.

Ultimately, I believe that mindset is the glue that will hold the other components together. Positivity will allow you to work through obstacles; however, once negativity enters your mind, you lose motivation and start falling off the path. Mindset is something that will keep appearing on your journey as you face new obstacles that stand between you and your goal, so it is important to ensure that a positive foundation is in place.

Chapter 3

YOUR WHY

"It's only after you've stepped outside your comfort zone that you begin to change, grow, and transform."
~Roy T. Bennett

I'm sure you've had people ask you WHY.
Why do you want to run a marathon?
Why do you want to get toned?
Why do you want to gain weight?
Why do you want to lose weight?
Why do you want to run around your yard?
Why do you pack your lunch?
Why do you stay up so late?
Why do you wake up so early?

Why? Why? Why? And the list can go on! Rather than looking at this one word as an annoying question, let's dig deeper and dissect the real reason WHY...according to YOU! The answer to this question has the ability to release so much energy, positivity, and enthusiasm into your mindset and how you view your journey, it's amazing!

As you might have noticed already, I have not defined the word "healthy". This is on purpose, in case you were wondering. Every woman (and man for that matter) on this Earth is an individual. It is impossible to define the word "healthy" in a personal sense that relates to every person. The word "healthy" can mean so many things, depending on the individual. It could mean getting through the day without pain, the ability to get off of a specific medication, lowering cholesterol, being able to be actively involved in the lives of loved ones, or maybe something totally different. Everyone is different. Everyone comes from different backgrounds. Heck, even though my sister and I grew up under the same roof, same ethnic background, same parents, same schools, same group of friends, we are as different as they come. I can tell you now, my definition of "healthy" is different, for both me and my sister, because we focus and work on different things that relate to our own lifestyle and personal issues.

I am not here to judge your "WHY" or define "Healthy" for you. We all come in different shapes and forms, have different starting points, and are gifted with different abilities. All of these differences should be celebrated. You have your own reason WHY for starting this journey. And that is the only WHY that matters. It will be the fuel that keeps you going throughout your journey.

It's Time To Reflect! I want you to take some time and think about these questions before you write out your WHY. Feel free to jot down notes next to the questions.

What are you trying to accomplish for yourself?

Who is important in your life?

What dreams or passions do you have?

What health issues do you have?

What might happen if you don't do anything about your health issues?

What is one thing you haven't been able to do in a while?

Now, it's time to write your WHY. Remember, there is no judgement. There is no wrong answer. This is YOUR answer, but the more elaborate and in depth you can go with your WHY the deeper roots it will have in creating your strength to keep on going and not giving up on yourself.

Why are YOU starting this journey?

Author's Note: As your journey progresses, YOUR WHY may change. That's okay! Don't be afraid to reevaluate as things change and goals are met. In all honesty, our journey never ends...it just gets readjusted. Use sticky notes to update your why and just stick them on this page so you can keep looking back at it as a reminder along the way.

Chapter 4

YOUR FINAL GOAL

"A Goal is a dream with a deadline." -Napoleon Hill

Congratulations! You now have a clearly defined WHY and now know why you are really on this journey to a healthy you. So many people do things for the wrong reasons, and you just figured out the RIGHT reason! You're off to a great start! It is now time to take that reason and apply it to form your final goal.

Your WHY will help you formulate your final goal on this journey. You may think I'm getting ahead of myself. The final goal sounds intimidating and scary. But, it is crucial to know where you want to be, in order to map out your path along the way. My dad loves planning. My childhood memory for every vacation we ever took was my dad mapping out our route and me helping him navigate. When I moved from Arizona to Michigan in 2017, he drove along with me and my three kids. Talk about wild and crazy. Before my husband and I even found a house to rent, he had started looking at maps and mapping my way from Arizona to Michigan. He wanted to know my address as soon as possible, so he could map out our route, rest stops, and hotels along the way....all in a timely manner. He would not let me use the GPS. Sure we had to add in extra stops for the kids and detour around some road construction, but that's life right? Our destination was still the same, we just had to adjust some things along the way in order to make it successful.

Your health journey is very similar. You need to know what your final destination is in order to plan and map out what you need to do to get there. It doesn't mean that the route is set in stone and you cannot stray from the plan. Life is crazy! Things change! Schedules change! My husband's work schedule was changing every two weeks...which meant my schedule changed every two weeks. Life changes! It's up to you to adapt and find alternate routes to get you to the same destination. It is very important to know that and to embrace that fact. Just because life throws us a detour doesn't mean we give up on the trip and turn around and go home. My new home was Michigan. I couldn't go back to Arizona. I had to find my way there, because my husband was waiting for me. Your new health and life is waiting for you. Don't give up on it just because an obstacle presents itself. It may take you longer, but you will still get there if you keep taking those detours and moving towards that final or long term goal.

It's Time To Reflect! Think about your WHY for starting this journey from the previous chapter. Let it help you formulate your final goal in your health journey.

What is my definition of healthy...according to ME?

What is my Final Goal for my health and fitness journey?

What is the <u>DATE</u> that I will aim to accomplish my final goal? (be honest and realistic with this date...things take time, so take that into consideration.)

What are some possible obstacles that I foresee standing in my way?

What are some short term goals, that I can celebrate, along the way to my Final Goal?

Notes and Additional Thoughts:

Notes and Additional Thoughts:

Author's Note: It is important to know that your final goal is not your final stop. It is the first destination of a lifetime of travel. You will continue to set new goals and improve upon yourself as you continue your new lifestyle. This initial goal is just to get you started on the right path in discovering "your" healthy.

Chapter 5

YOUR SELF-TALK

"I am the greatest. I said that even before I knew I was." -Muhammad Ali

Let me just bring something to your attention. If you've gotten this far in the book already, and you've completed all of the reflection portions, you have already started building a solid foundation for your long-term success. You, my friend, have officially planted roots and put meaning to your transformation. You have figured out whether you have a positive or negative mindset and what you need to work on. You have figured out the roots of WHY you are even on this journey. And you've figured out your exact goal and the date by which you want to achieve this goal. Can you believe you've done all of that already? Those things seem so easy, but those are the deep questions and concepts that you need to have a solid grasp on before continuing. You should be proud and celebrate those small, yet necessary accomplishments.

But we can't stop there. Now, it's time to figure out how to get to that goal by putting meaningful actions into motion. Along the lines of a positive mindset, self-talk will either encourage us to move forward or discourage us and stop us from progressing forward. If during the earlier chapters, you've discovered that you have a positive mindset, then I hope that you take my challenge after this section and see if you are already incorporating these things into your life. If you discovered that you're not as positive as you thought you were, I will provide you with some techniques and ideas that you can choose to incorporate into your life to help create a more positive self-talk habit.

What is self-talk? Self-talk are the words we think to ourselves or say to ourselves, about ourselves, throughout the day. If you have a negative self-talk, you may find yourself discouraging yourself or talking yourself out of things. Negative self-talk may sound like this, "I'm never going to make my goal anyway, so why am I even trying." "Ugh, I failed again." "I hate how this outfit looks on me." "I'm just going to give up, because no one thinks I can anyway."

Positive self-talk sounds more like, "Okay...this was a stressful day, but I have 10 minutes while the kids are playing nicely to get in a short workout so I can keep moving forward." "I got this!" "I may have failed this attempt, but I'll get it next time." "I will reach my goal." "I am beautiful." "I am worth it." "I'm an awesome mother." "I'm an awesome friend." "I'm just plain AWESOME!"

Do you see the difference? Do you see how one is a total bummer, while the other one is really motivating and encouraging? You may think that if you have a positive self-talk that you sound boastful or arrogant. But guess what? These are your thoughts! No one is listening to your thoughts. So you won't seem arrogant or boastful. But to set the record straight, you ARE allowed to say those things about yourself too! Who cares what anyone else thinks? Don't let anyone else's negativity cloud up your accomplishments and success. It's okay to acknowledge things you're good at.

Your self-talk will either encourage you or discourage you. In order to move forward on your health and fitness journey, you need to learn how to change any negativity to positivity. We will work on putting a positive spin on any situation, no matter how bad you think it may be. This is NOT easy! It takes practice! It takes TIME! Which is why I will be challenging you to put it into practice for 21 days in a row. Who is to say you can't? Who is to say that you aren't good enough? You are good enough! You can do anything you put your mind to! And the more you keep telling yourself that with positive self-talk, it won't matter who puts you down, because deep inside you will still know that you are worth it and you WILL achieve what you set out to achieve. Are you ready?!

It's Time To Reflect! I'm going to allow you to reflect first, before I give you some answers. This journey is about looking at yourself and your life. I want you to dig deep and find positive things to say about yourself.

What are my strengths?

How does my favorite outfit make me feel?

How do I help people?

What do I do for my kids?

What do I do for my fur babies?

Now that you have discovered some things that make you feel good and realize that you are wonderful, **List some phrases (in the space below) that you can say about yourself or to yourself that are positive and encouraging.**

If you are struggling to come up with anything nice to say about yourself, I'm here to help. Remember, now is not the time to be modest. Now is the time to get your mind in the game and kick butt. Show others what you're made of and how awesome you are! So below I have some examples of phrases that you can say to yourself daily and some ideas of where to find some inspiration if you are really struggling. There are no excuses! There is always a way that you can work on your mindset and self-talk. PRACTICE!

I like to think that I have somewhat mastered this concept; however, I am constantly reminded that I have not. Life gets tough. Things happen and obstacles try to pull me down. But instead of getting stuck in a rut, practicing positive self-talk has helped me learn the tools to use in order to bounce back more quickly and get my mindset right again, so I don't totally fall off from my goals. This challenge and activity isn't the fix all, end all. It is simply a strategy to use and practice for when life throws us lemons. We take those lemons and make it lemonade or spice up our water with it. Don't sell yourself short. Be patient with yourself and give yourself time to remind yourself that you are capable and worthy of reaching your goals set for yourself.

The Positive Self-Talk Toolbox:

Morning Positive Self-Talk Phrases:

* "My hair looks great today!"

* "I am going to try my best today."

* "I am going to smile at everyone today."

* "I got this!"

* "I will make healthy choices today."

* "I am an awesome woman/mother/wife/daughter/ grandma!"

* "I am beautiful."

* "I am worth it!"

* "I am rockin this outfit!"

* "I am going to do amazing things today!"

Evening Positive Self-Talk Phrases:

* "I did my best today."

* "I don't need praise from anyone else, I know I rocked it today."

* "I am proud of myself."

19

* "I may not have done my best, but tomorrow is a new day and I will try again tomorrow."

* "I think I impacted someone's life today."

* "I did it!"

* "I will not give up."

* "I am making things happen!"

What can I do if I'm just struggling with telling myself positive things?

1. Look to a favorite song or poem that inspires you or gets you in a more positive mood.

2. Read a chapter from an inspirational book.

3. Google motivational quotes.

4. Reread your WHY and your goal.

5. Look back at the reflection questions and think about all the things you do for the ones you love.

Hopefully you now have a good grasp on what positive self-talk is and what you can say to yourself to help keep you positive and proud of yourself. Now, let's work on incorporating it into your daily routine.

For the next 21 days, you will work on using the list you created and incorporate at least 1 positive self-talk phrase into your day. I don't care if you need to write it on a sticky note and stick it to your mirror in the morning and read it while you're drying your hair or brushing your teeth. Use one of those fancy mirror markers. I have even seen some positive mirror decals with cute phrases like, "You Are Amazing" and "You are Beautiful", that you can put on your mirror in a neat and classy way. Saying those simple words out loud have more of an impact than we think. You'll find that if you start saying these phrases to yourself, then over the next 21 days it won't feel like a chore anymore and you'll actually start thinking more positive thoughts on your own without even having to look at the saying. Whatever way you use to remember, do it! You might even want to create a positive quote wallpaper background for your phone. Whatever works. For 21 days!

The challenge starts on the next page…Ready….GO!

21 Day Positive Self-Talk Challenge

My WHY:

_____

My GOAL:

_____

START DATE: _____   END DATE: _____

Check off the box when you complete each day. Next to the day, write the phrase you said to yourself that kept you positive for that day.

☐ Day 1:

_____

☐ Day 2:

_____

☐ Day 3:

_____

☐ Day 4:

_____

☐ Day 5:

_____

☐ Day 6:

_____

☐ Day 7:

_____

You have completed a week of positive self-talk! You rock!

What were some of the negative thoughts that kept creeping into mind? (This will help you be more aware of them and try to find phrases that will help you overcome those negative thoughts.)

Bring on the next 7 days!!! YOU GOT THIS!

☐ Day 8:

_____

☐ Day 9:

_____

☐ Day 10:

_____

☐ Day 11:

_____

☐ Day 12:

_____

☐ Day 13:

_____

☐ Day 14:

_____

You've completed the next 7 days!!! Awesome job! Are you getting the hang of it? Do you still have to look at your sticky notes? Are you catching yourself lifting yourself up in tough times without even trying anymore? Either way…Keep on going! You're doing great so far! You are transforming! Don't Quit! Only 7 Days left in this Challenge!

☐ Day 15:

_____

☐ Day 16:

_____

☐ Day 17:

_____

☐ Day 18:

_____

☐ Day 19:

_____

☐ Day 20:

_____

☐ Day 21:

_____

WOOHOO!!! You have completed the 21 days of Positive Self-Talk Challenge! You should be so proud of yourself!

How do you feel? Are you becoming more positive towards yourself? If not, don't be afraid to go through it again until you have a better grasp. We all run at different speeds. That's why YOU are in control. Don't feel bad about going at a slower pace. As long as you are genuinely working on it, then you will start to feel a transformation on the inside and you are on your way to a healthy you. In all honesty, this is something I work on daily. It is something you will continue to work on as well throughout your health and fitness journey.

Author's Note: I'd love to hear that you have completed the 21 day Positive Self-Talk Challenge and how it has effected you. Feel free to e-mail me so we can celebrate together! katy.katydidfitness@gmail.com

Chapter 6

YOUR SELF-IMAGE

"I was always looking outside myself for strength and confidence, but it comes from within. It is there all of the time." -Anna Freud

I believe that self-image is an extremely important topic that impacts a lot of women on a daily basis. Self-Image is the mental image you have about yourself. This can affect your self-esteem and confidence.

A lot of times we base our self-image on how we compare ourselves to other people that are completely different than us, with things that we really have no control over, like height, and body type. I am completely guilty of this as you will soon find out. It's human nature to compare and observe, but we need to be careful about what we are actually comparing.

Many times, the comparison makes us wish that we were completely different, which will cause us to be dissatisfied with ourselves, leading to a negative self-image. We don't even realize that there are realistic changes that we can make that are within the parameters of our body compositions that will ultimately improve our self-image and keep us striving towards our health and fitness goals.

Let me share a little story with you. I had mentioned earlier that my sister and I are practically polar opposites. In addition to the complete personality difference, she has blonde hair blue eyes, I have brown hair brown eyes. She is taller than me and has a slim and linear build, and I am short, curvy, and muscular. She could eat whatever she wanted all the time, I always felt like I was on a diet to just maintain my size. As a younger sister, all I wanted to do was be skinny like my older sister. I felt fat.

At the time, I didn't realize that I was comparing apples to oranges. I didn't realize that I was a totally different body type than her and that I couldn't change that. My sister's body type is an ectomorph, which means that she has a slim and lean physique with some light muscular tone. I, on the other hand, am a mesomorph, which means that I am more muscular and am able to gain muscle more easily than the other body types. I will go into more detail about the body types in a bit, but the point is, I didn't know the things I know now about each body type. I didn't realize that I stored fat in different places than her. I didn't realize that I gain and lose weight differently than her. I didn't realize that even the food I ate processed differently in my body, than hers.

And because of this lack of knowledge, I became very critical with myself. That personal battle gave me a negative mind-set and instilled a lot of negative self-talk. I wished I was something I was not; I strived to be a body type that I could never achieve...slender and linear. Instead, I was muscular and curvy, but I never embraced it. I didn't like my shape, because I associated it with looking fat.

It wasn't until after college and I moved to Las Vegas, when I realized I was doing things all wrong. I walked into 24 Hour Fitness and hopped on the treadmill for my cardio session and observed a beautiful mesomorphic, fitness competitor across the gym, practicing her walk and posing on stage where they do classes in the gym. I really admired her. Granted, she was taller than me and had long blonde hair, but she had the muscular physique that I struggled with having for so long. She presented herself as muscular and confident. It wasn't until then, that I realized a muscular build could be beautiful too. From that moment, my self-image began to shift into something more positive for myself. I finally realized that I could enhance my muscularity and work on my physique to enhance my qualities rather than try to hide them. Yes, it took me 22 years to figure this all out about myself. Better late than never!

Here's a fun little fact. After moving to Arizona, four years later and finally entering my very first figure competition, that same girl that I watched for years at the gym in Vegas, was presenting the awards! My husband saw her and knew I was acting like a giddy school girl. I had gotten 2nd place and she presented my award to me! She had no clue the impact she had on me and my self-image transformation. She was one of the reasons why I even thought to be on that stage.

It took me a long time to embrace my muscular physique and build a positive image of myself, but the important thing is that I did. I train to compliment my body. Now, it doesn't matter what anyone thinks of me. Someone is always going to have an opinion. I will not let anyone else's opinion effect my positive self-image of myself.

One thing that I learned is that no body type is better than the other. Each body type can gain fat and lose fat. Today, I challenge you to look at yourself. I challenge you to figure out your own body type if you do not know already. In the reflection section, I will define and explain what each one is. Once you figure out your own body type, no longer compare yourself to someone that is created completely different than you. That always ends with disappointment. Instead, learn how you can best exercise and eat according to your own body type, so you can discover the healthy you that you are striving for. I truly believe that is one of the big secrets that will keep you moving forward.

It's Time To Reflect!   When you look in the mirror, your first instinct may be picking out all the things that are wrong with your body.   We are going to work on finding the positive!   It's time to improve your self-image!

Let's figure out what body type you are.

If you are an Ectomorph, you have a slim and linear build.   You have a lean physique and light musculature. You enjoy cardio and may participate in jogging/running events currently.   It is also difficult for you to build muscle.

If you are a Mesomorph, you have more of an athletic build. You have an athletic build and have the ability to gain muscle more easily.

If you are an Endomorph, you have a heavier rounded body build.   You have the ability to gain fat easily if you're not careful.   You typically do not partake in any cardio activities unless absolutely necessary.

Here's a tip…If you're not sure what type you are, look back to younger pictures of yourself.   Then see where you fit.   Our bone structure stays the same, we just gain and lose weight and muscle definition as years progress.

Like I mentioned before, and it's worth repeating, by no means is one body type better than the other. Each body type has the ability to become unhealthy, as well as, the ability to achieve great health and fitness goals. Each of these types can be extremely successful, but it is important to be aware of which one you are, because it opens your eyes to how you will want to approach your exercise, and nutrition. Yes, your body type can matter in these areas, but it doesn't limit your success to discovering a healthy you. So it's time to take off the blinders and figure out which one you are, so we can continue moving in the right direction.

Are you an ectomorph, mesomorph, or endomorph?

Now that you know your body type, write down what you love about your body.

What does your husband/boyfriend/partner love about your body?

What is your favorite body part?

31

Take a look at your body. Think about your favorite body part and what others love about your body. Now write down some ways you would improve your body, so you can enhance the things you love.

I will be addressing how your body type will effect your fitness and nutrition throughout the book, but for now, congratulations on discovering what YOUR body type is, embracing it, and committing to improve yourself in discovering a healthy you! I'm proud of you! Now, let's get exercising!

Chapter 7

SCHEDULING YOUR TIME

"We learn wisdom from failure much more than success. We often discover what we will do, by finding out what we will not do." -Samuel Smiles

You are ready! You are mentally prepared to take on your goal wholeheartedly. Now, the next obstacle... scheduling everything. An excuse I hear more than I can count is, "I don't have time to exercise." "I'm too busy." "I work." "I'm in school." "I don't have time to myself." No matter what you do in your day, you have the same 24 hours as everyone else. It's how you utilize that time. If you find yourself saying these things to yourself or others, it's not that you don't have enough time. The reality is, you weren't all in before. You were not mentally prepared to take on this journey yet, so the excuses surface and other things took priority, leaving you without time. Think about it. Am I right? Sometimes it's a hard truth to accept, but we prioritize things that we view as important first. And most women don't have themselves at the top of that list. Which means any activity related to themselves ends up being at the bottom of the "if I have time left" section...which, let's face it...never gets accomplished.

But that is all different now! If you've completed the chapters up until this point you are now mentally prepared to take on this journey. You are ready to give yourself a chance. I will show you how to prioritize your day differently. It's amazing how many things you can get done, if you actually value the tasks and take a little time to plan.

The first thing you need to do is to write down your daily routine. Write down everything you do from breakfast to bedtime. For the most part, our weeks are very similar, but our daily routine can vary depending on certain activities like soccer practice, dance class, or school. If your days change often, write down all your possible routines based on the schedule you have. For example, you might have a child in soccer on Wednesdays and Fridays. Your routine for those days may look different than your routine on Monday and Tuesday when you do not have to drive to soccer practice. Make sure each routine is separated. Don't generalize. Be as specific as possible.

Let's take action! On the next page, I have provided you with a template to write down your daily routines. Take this template and create your own table in a notebook or journal and create 4 sections for 4 different possible routines that you may have throughout your week, depending on your life. If you have more routines, then add more columns. For each routine, write down the days in which you follow this routine. This will help you stay organized as you plan your time.

Possible Daily Schedules

	Routine 1 Days I use this routine: ___	Routine 2 Days I use this routine: ___	Routine 3 Days I use this routine: ___	Routine 4 Days I use this routine: ___
5:00-6:00am				
6:00-7:00				
7:00-8:00				
8:00-9:00				
9:00-10:00				
10:00-11:00				
11:00-12 pm				
12:00-1:00				
1:00-2:00				

	Routine 1 Days I use this routine: ___	Routine 2 Days I use this routine: ___	Routine 3 Days I use this routine: ___	Routine 4 Days I use this routine: ___
2:00-3:00				
3:00-4:00				
4:00-5:00				
5:00-6:00				
6:00-7:00				
8:00-9:00				
9:00-10:00				
10:00-11:00				
11:00-12am				

Great work! You can now actually see your daily routines on paper. Now, go get a different color marker or highlighter or anything that stands out. Look at each routine you have. Highlight the blank spots on your chart. Pay attention to what days they fall under. After highlighting all of the blank areas on your chart, try to find one 30 minute block of time somewhere in your routine and write WORKOUT in that spot. Make sure to star it or circle it.

If you don't have time to fit something in, there has to be some wiggle room in your schedule somewhere. Look for a 10-20 minute block of time.

You may have laundry or vacuuming listed every day. Yes, that is a task we find ourselves doing daily, but it is okay to skip a day or squeeze in a workout during that time. I end up doing laundry throughout the day, around all the other tasks I need to get done anyway, so why not work around a workout too. It's possible. Take a look again to see if there are any tasks like this, that you can be a little more lenient with and find some wiggle room. You can get a lot done in 10-30 minutes if you try.

Do you see a pattern of when you wrote WORKOUT? Do you find similarities in the time of day that you have some free time? Are times drastically different with each daily routine? These are all things to be aware of. Sometimes we think that if one day doesn't work, we just scrap even trying on other days, when reality the open time slot we have is just different.

Let me also point out that there may actually be a daily routine that is just too busy for you. And that's okay! But as long as you wrote WORKOUT somewhere, you have something to work with during the week and can have success. If you cannot find a single spot in any of your daily routines to write WORKOUT, then you need to reevaluate your routines and see how you can give yourself some time for your health. Isn't it up to us to stay healthy, so we can take care of everyone else? What happens when we get run down and sick and out of commission? The house falls apart. You are the glue that keeps everything running smoothly. That's why we are so darn tired! But it's so important for us to stay healthy. It's so important to find that time for your health, and exercise is an important part of that.

What time did you write WORKOUT on your chart?

Routine 1 _____

Routine 2 _____

Routine 3 _____

Routine 4 _____

You may have just found the previous question really difficult. Hang on to your hat, because I'm going to challenge you even further.

Pick a different highlighter color or pen color, and take a look at your routine again. Try to find another 10-30 minute block of time for each routine and write WORKOUT in that section AGAIN. WHAT?!?! I promise, I'm not trying to sabotage you.

If you were able to do this, Great work!!! If not, that's okay! Just because you couldn't do this portion doesn't mean you will fail. Let me tell you why I challenged you. Writing down at least 2 blocks of time for each daily routine allows you to have a time to fall back on in case something comes up and you aren't able to get your workout in during your allotted time. I mean work schedules change... kids don't nap... things happen. I DO NOT want you to work out twice in a day! NOT AT ALL! This task is a way to have a back up plan, in case something comes up. I'm trying to set you up for success, not failure. So now that you know the method behind my madness, can you go back to your routines and find a 30 minute back up spot somewhere in one of your routines? Go ahead and try.

You just completed a task that very few people actually do. It's time to practice some positive self-talk, because you are rocking it! You wrote down your busy schedule and you were able to pick out at least one 30 minute block of time in your daily routine. That's something to celebrate!

We aren't done yet. Days turn into weeks and that can get really overwhelming at times. Like I said before, it is not necessary to workout during every single opening in which you wrote WORKOUT on your daily routine. I recommend to start working out at least 3 days a week. If you are brand new and overwhelmed, then pick 1 or 2 days to start with. Working your way up to 3 might be a goal. The key is to pick a number that doesn't overwhelm and that you can be consistent with.

I am an avid lifter, but I definitely didn't keep my lifting routine throughout each of my 3 pregnancies. I gained 35-40 pounds with each pregnancy. After each child, it was a total readjustment all over again, but I took the steps that I'm sharing with you, and worked my way through it. After my third baby, Lincoln, was born, I actually had to start with 1 day a week, because I was so overwhelmed with managing 2 kids and a newborn, it took me a while to actually figure out a routine that worked for me. I eventually worked my way up to 3 days and now I work out 5 -6 days a week.

It's okay to start slow. It's okay to move faster if you feel you have a good grasp on your routine. To avoid burn out or quitting, rather than stopping completely, you want to simply back off on the number of days you exercise, until you get into a good routine again.

With that said, you are now going to decide how many days a week you want to start exercising and decide what days will work best for you.

In the chart below, pick the days that will work best for your workouts based on your daily routines. Write the time period in which you will workout. It should match your opening on the routine that works for you.

On the following chart, you will see my example of how I figured out my schedule to start working out. Tuesdays I follow my Routine 1 daily schedule. I have an opening to workout from 11-11:30am. Thursday my day follows Routine 2 and I can workout best at 2-3pm. And Saturday I follow my Routine 4 schedule and can workout from 7-8pm. My Routine 3 schedule is just too crazy for me to workout at all, so I skip it. After mapping my schedule, I now know that I can workout on Tuesdays from 11-11:30am, Thursdays from 2-3pm, and Saturdays from 7-8pm.

Example:
Best Days/Times To Workout

	Routine 1	Routine 2	Routine 3	Routine 4
Sunday				
Monday				
Tuesday	Workout 11-11:30 am			
Wednesday				
Thursday		Workout 2-3pm		
Friday				
Saturday				Workout 7-8pm

It's Time To Reflect! It's your turn! Flip back to your daily routines and try to fill in your chart below.

YOUR Best Days/Times To Workout

	Routine 1	Routine 2	Routine 3	Routine 4
Sunday				
Monday				
Tuesday				
Wednesday				
Thursday				
Friday				
Saturday				

I will work out _____ days per week.

I will work out (circle what applies):
Morning, Afternoon, Evening

These are the days that work best for me.

Congratulations! You now have a solid grasp of how many days you can handle workouts during the week and you know which days they actually are!

Knowing this is a huge breakthrough. Scheduling it into your routine will make a huge difference in actually getting it done. I personally write my workout schedule on my white board calendar in my kitchen. That is where I put all my important events that I can't forget. Having a visual reminder will mentally prepare you for your workout on those days, rather than basing your workout on your energy level and how you think you feel that day. You'll be amazed how differently you look at a workout when you add a little more value to it by writing it in a place with other important events.

Chapter 8

EXERCISE ACCORDING TO YOUR GOAL

"Our greatest weakness lies in giving up. The most certain way to succeed is to always try just one more time." -Thomas Edison

I'm sure you've seen a lot of magazines, blogs, and books on exercise already. You know the one's I'm talking about...the ones that promise extreme results in a short amount of time. Don't let these titles fool you. Yes, they may be effective, but not without a very strict mindset, routine, and nutrition plan...and consistency. Consistency is the key to exercise. If you are not consistent with any exercise, then you can't expect to see any results. Even if you are really consistent for one week, then you stop the next...that is not being consistent. Consistency means that you are continuing this routine for a long period of time. Also, just like diets, not all exercises work for everyone. It is important to find the exercises that will get you closer to your personal goals.

I will talk more about nutrition in the upcoming chapters, but even if you aren't worried about your nutrition now, eventually, you will need to take a look at it. You'll find your progress has plateaued even with exercise. That is when you need to look at nutrition. This works the other way around as well. You may only be focusing on nutrition and not exercise, but you'll get to a point where you feel stuck and then you need to start incorporating exercise. So rather than focusing on just one, you will get better results if you can work on both, simultaneously. However, it is not necessary if you are struggling with both. They both will come into play eventually, but the important thing is to be able to be consistent with whatever you are working on at the time.

Exercise is important, because it can provide you with the *mobility*, *strength*, *agility*, *cardiovascular health*, *weight-loss*, and *joint health* that you may need in your day-to-day life. Think about these words. After reading all of those goals, one of the words probably stuck out to you, because it applies to your personal goal.

Which Words Stuck Out At You?

If *mobility* stuck out, then you may have tightened tendons and ligaments that need stretched, so you are able to increase your range of motion. Spending more time stretching specific areas will help in this area. Flexibility exercises will also help increase your range of motion.

If *strength* stuck out to you, you may either want to tone up or even build some muscle. This type of exercise includes body weight exercises and weight training. Body weight exercises are great to get started and still see results, but if they become easy for you, then you need to add resistance through resistance bands, ankle weights, weighted plates, medicine balls, dumbbells, anything with some added weight. I also would like to be clear about something...and I get this a lot. Working out with weights will not make you "bulky". In order to gain a lot of muscle you need to lift with fewer repetitions and heavier weights. I just want to make sure we are clear in the fact that the equipment will not make you "bulky" or extremely muscular; it's how you use the equipment. It is all goal oriented in which you can control.

If *agility* stuck out to you, then you want to work on your speed and quickness. You may want to incorporate some sprints, ladder drills, and even explosive squat jumps into your routine.

If *cardiovascular health* stuck out to you, then you are trying to increase your endurance. To raise your endurance takes practice. This takes a variety of cardio or aerobic exercises. I recommend you choose one that you enjoy, because if you don't enjoy it, then you will want to quit. Swimming, biking, walking, jogging, running, dancing, different cardio machines are all great ways to practice and increase your endurance. Another tip I recommend is to start small. Know your limitations with distance or time and start there, then slowly increase as you feel it getting easier. It will get easier, it just takes consistency.

If *weight-loss* stuck out to you, then you are probably aiming to burn fat. You can do this with a mixture of all different exercises combined. I hate to burst your bubble, but unfortunately you cannot decide the location in which your body loses fat. That is all dependent on your body and how you gain and lose weight. For example, I gain weight in my hips and butt first. On the other hand, I lose weight from my upper body first and melt down like a candle. So, my hips and legs are the last thing to lose, but first to gain. You should know these things about your own body.

How do you gain and lose weight?

Knowing this will make you more aware of the overall changes happening to your body rather than focusing in on that one stubborn area that isn't changing.

Weight-loss can be achieved with any of the previous topics. You can mix and match the areas that interest you and incorporate them in a way where you are raising your heart rate in order to burn fat. For example. Wanting to lose weight and tone up. Well, in order to achieve that, I like to incorporate cardio, whether that is something you enjoy or agility exercises, and strength, which is the bodyweight and weighted exercises to firm your muscles, in a way that raises your heart rate. You can do this by incorporating supersets, or circuits with the bodyweight exercises and weights. There are so many different varieties and ways in which to achieve this goal, so please, if you have any concerns or questions please don't hesitate to e-mail me at katy@katydidfitness.com. I would love to chat with you and help guide you further.

Finally, if *joint health* stuck out to you, you may have some health issues that you need to work around. Whether it is Arthritis, osteoarthritis, or an injury, flexibility, strength, and aerobic exercises are good to incorporate into your routine. Moving the joints through flexibility exercises increases the lubrication over the cartilage and joint space. The movement helps increase blood flow to the area and helps reduce joint swelling. Low impact strength training exercises help strengthen the muscles around the joints for better stability. And low impact cardio exercises like swimming and cycling provide movement for the joints without great impact and help increase cardiovascular health as well.

It's Time To Reflect: Reflecting on your goals and health issues will give you a better idea of how you should be exercising.

What area would you like to improve: *mobility* (range of motion), *strength* (tone or build muscle), *agility* (speed), *cardiovascular health* (endurance), *weight-loss* or *joint health* (low impact)**?**

What health issues do you have?

It is always important to make sure you consult your doctor before taking on any exercise routine. Your doctor may set some restrictions on your exercise, but that's okay. Exercise can always be modified in some way.

Congratulations! You have come so far. You have now specified the exercise that coincide with your health and fitness goal and are ready to put it all into action.   Great work!   I will show you how to do just that in the next chapter!

Chapter 9

CREATING YOUR WORKOUT

"If something stands between you and your success, move it. Never be denied."
-Dwayne "The Rock" Johnson, professional wrestler and actor

There's nothing like a little motivation from "The Rock" with this quote. I know he motivates me! Now that you're motivated and ready to get to work, I am going to walk you through how to create your own workout according to the fitness goals you wrote down in the previous chapter.

That's right! By the end of this chapter you will have a workout routine that you can start incorporating into your schedule. You will know what type of exercises you should be doing, as well as, knowing how to switch things up in order to make things easier or more challenging as you progress.

Keep in mind that these exercises are not where you should end your journey. These templates, that I am about to give you, are just to get you started in creating appropriate workout habits for your specific goals. Don't be afraid to keep learning and adding exercises to your list. Eventually, you may be interested in checking out KatydidFitness.com, where I provide you with other body specific exercise ideas that you may be interested in trying. I am here to guide you the whole way, whether it's through this book, e-mail, or chatting through my Katydid Fitness mobile app. I'm devoted to a healthy you!

Now, I assume you have checked with your doctor and are cleared to workout. If not, make sure to do that as soon as possible! Look back at the previous chapter and get a good idea of what category goal you will be targeting: *mobility, strength, agility, cardiovascular health, weigh-loss,* or *joint health*.

I will be providing you with some awesome workout templates for each goal. To save space and to keep things moving, I provide an index, in the back of this book, explaining how to perform each exercise.

It's time to get out that highlighter or pen and star the exercise goal list you will be focusing on. Focus on that section only! I know it will be tempting to skim through and see if each goal is different or not. Now that I said that, I know you will flip through and look. Do what you must, but I assure you they are completely different, and if you start looking through and wondering if you should be doing something different, you will lose sight of your goal and try to fit your goal into an area where it doesn't fit.

Don't lose sight of your goal and your WHY! Those are the two most important things to remember throughout your journey. Once you accomplish your current goal, you are encouraged to come back to this chapter and create a new workout according to a new goal. But for now, don't confuse yourself and give yourself more work than I'm already giving you. Save your energy for the actual workout!

Before we start, I do want to clarify the difference between a strength goal and a weight-loss goal.

* If you are happy with your weight, but want to strengthen and tone, then you can flip to the STRENGTH EXERCISES section.

* If you have weight that you still want to lose, but also want to firm, strengthen, and tone what is underneath, then I suggest you skip to the WEIGHT-LOSS section!!!

Okay! Are You Ready?! Take a deep breath!

Go ahead and find the exercise goal list that applies to you and let's get started!

Mobility Exercises

Chest Exercises:
* Kneeling Thoracic Rotation
* Chest Stretch Standing
* Floor Chest Stretch

Abdominal Exercises:
* Rotating Lower Body
* Bent Leg Core Rotation Lying
* Single Leg Dynamic Stretch

Arm Exercises:
* Seated Arm Shake-SHOULDER, BICEP, TRICEP
* Tricep Stretch Behind Back-TRICEP
* Single Arm Tricep Stretch-TRICEP
* Bicep Stretch Standing-BICEP

Back/Shoulder/Neck Exercises:
* W-Pump- UPPER BACK, SHOULDERS
* Eagle Supine- LOWER BACK
* Neck Stretch Sideways- NECK
* Windmill-BACK, SHOULDERS

Leg Exercises:
* Ankle Mobilization Seated
* Heel To Toe
* Leg Swings Front and Back
* Leg Swing Sideways
* Bent Over Toe Touch

Mobility Exercises (continued)

Low Impact Cardio:
* Swimming
* Yoga
* Walking
* Bicycle

Remember these exercises are explained in the index in the back of the book. In addition to these exercises, you can also use a foam roller to help loosen up your muscles before and after you do your exercises. Loosening your muscles before exercises will help you reach full range of motion during the exercise, which in turn will increase your mobility.

It takes time and consistency to increase flexibility. Mobility workouts are meant to be performed at a slower pace with focus on stretching and reaching full range of motion. Don't rush! Also, don't forget to relax and loosen the muscles with a warm bath as well.

Once you feel your mobility has improved and are comfortable, you may want to start incorporating some low impact joint health workouts into your routine.

It's Your Turn To Take ACTION!!! Your goal is **_mobility_**! Here are templates to help you create different workouts that you will be able to insert into your weekly routine.

1. Look at the templates.

2. Fill in an exercise from the list above in the template for the appropriate body part.

3. Circle whether you want to hold the exercise for 10 seconds or do 10 repetitions for the exercise.

Mobility Workout 1
Upper Body

Body Part	Exercise for the body part	Sets	Time or Reps	Rest (seconds)
Warm Up	March in place	1	3 min	60
Chest		2	10 sec or 10 rep	60
Back		2	10 sec or 10 rep	60
Tricep		2	10 sec	60
Bicep		2	10sec or 10 rep	60
Back or Neck		2	10sec or 10 rep	60
Shoulders		2	10 rep	60
CARDIO		1	15 min	90

This particular workout focuses on your upper body. This workout is okay to do once a week. You want to eventually work your whole body throughout the week, so you will want to assign this workout for 1 day and rotate it in with lower body and core workouts that are to follow.

As you become more familiar with different mobility exercises, you may want to add your own exercises to the list and insert them into future upper body workouts that you create to switch things up.

Great Work! You are off to a great start in learning how to create your own workouts. Let's go for Workout 2!

Mobility Workout 2
Lower Body

Body Part	Exercise for the body part	Sets	Time or Rep	Rest (seconds)
Warm Up	March in place	1	3 min	60
Leg		2	10 sec or 10 rep	60
Leg		2	10 sec or 10 rep	60
Leg		2	10 sec	60
Calf		2	10 sec or 10 rep	60
CARDIO		1	20 min	90

This workout focuses on your lower body. This workout is okay to do once a week. Once again, you eventually want to work your whole body throughout the week, so you will want to assign this workout for 1 day and rotate it through with upper body and core workouts.

The reasoning behind splitting up upper and lower body is for a few practical reasons:

1. It creates a shorter workout that you can insert into your day easily.

2. It allows you to focus on a specific area, so you can work out with intention and aim for mobility in specific locations.

3. It also allows each area to rest during the days the other areas are worked. It is important to allow for rest, which many people feel they do not need. So, this gives you the rest in those muscles and ligaments while working other areas.

Mobility Workout 3
Core

Body Part	Exercise for the body part	Sets	Time or Rep	Rest (seconds)
Warm Up	March in place	1	3 min	60
Abs		2	10 sec or 10 rep	60
Back		2	10 sec or 10 rep	60
Abs		2	10 sec	60
Back		2	10sec or 10 rep	60
CARDIO		1	20 min	90

This workout focuses on your core mobility. When I talk about core, you may assume that means your ab muscles. But in reality, it also focuses on our lower back because that is the opposing muscle group. If you have pain in one area, it could mean that you are weak or tight in the opposing muscle group, because you are compensating somehow for the weak area which puts strain on the stronger area.

Assign this workout 1 time a week. Rotate this core workout with the upper body and lower body workout throughout the week. As you become more familiar with different mobility exercises, you may want to add more core exercises to the list and insert them into future workouts to switch things up.

Workout Option 4
FULL BODY

Body Part	Exercise for the body part	Sets	Time or Rep	Rest (seconds)
Warm Up	March in place	1	3 min	60
Chest		2	10 sec or 10 rep	60
Back		2	10 sec or 10 rep	60
Tricep		2	10 sec	60
Bicep		2	10 sec or 10 rep	60
Back or Neck		2	10 sec or 10 rep	60
Shoulders		2	10 rep	60
Legs		2	10 rep	60
Abs		2	10 rep	60
CARDIO		1	10 min	90

This workout focuses on the whole body. If you had trouble figuring out when to fit in a workout into your schedule, you may want to consider doing a full body workout 1 or 2 times a week, because you do not have enough time during the week to rotate through the separate body parts. That's okay. Remember, anything is better than nothing. Make it work for you! You have options. You decide what works best for you.

You may want to use this template to create a couple full body workouts with some different exercises to keep things different on the days you do have time to work out.

If you are able to work out more than 3 times a week, then you can definitely add this workout into the rotation at the end of your body part split workouts!

Ways You Can Adjust These Workouts:

1. If the workout takes too long, only do 1 set of each exercise or trim the cardio by 5 minutes.

2. If the workout is too short, the you can add 1 set to each exercise.

3. If the workout is too hard, you can hold the exercise for as long as you can or do as many repetitions as you can and work your way up to 10.

4. If the workout is too easy, you can increase the length that you hold the exercise (no need to go past 30 seconds) or perform the exercise for 15-20 repetitions.

5. Take more rest if you need it, but remember not to go too fast through the rest period.   You are focusing on the stretch and range of motion.   It's not a weight-loss circuit.

6. Finally, if you can do 20 repetitions with ease after 2 sets and you are feeling more flexible and mobile, then it is time to start creating workouts in the LOW-IMPACT JOINT HEALTH section.

You Did It! You just wrote yourself a mobility workout routine according to YOU! You can now work out with a purpose and a goal in mind, rather than just working out on a feeling or whim! WAY TO GO!

I can't wait for you to put this to action in the next chapter.   When you are ready, you can head on over to **Chapter 10**!

That is where the real fun will begin!

Strength Exercises

Abdominal Exercises:
* Oblique Crunch- OBLIQUES
* Russian Twist- OBLIQUES
* Bicycle Crunch- OBLIQUES
* Double Crunch- ALL ABS
* Lying Toe Touch- ALL ABS
* Reverse Crunch- LOWER ABS
* Lying Leg Raises- LOWER ABS

Bicep Exercises:
* Alternating Bicep Curls
* Concentration Curls
* Alternating Hammer Curls
* Seated Double Bicep Curls
* Seated Double Hammer Curls

Tricep Exercises:
* Tricep Dip With Legs Extended
* Close Push-Ups
* Close Push-Ups On Knees
* Seated Tricep Extension
* Chair Dips With Bent Legs
* Chair Dips With Legs Elevated
* Tricep Kickbacks

Strength Exercises (continued)

Back Exercises:
* Superman- LOWER BACK, GLUTES, SHOULDERS
* Reverse Fly- UPPER BACK
* Bent Over Rows- UPPER BACK
* Reverse Grip Bent Over Rows- BACK
* Bird Dog Alternating- BACK, ABS
* Hyperextension Using Exercise Ball- LOWER BACK
* Plank- BACK, ABS, CHEST

Chest Exercises:
* Push-Up
* Push-Up On Knees
* Wide Push-Up
* Decline Push-Up
* Incline Push-Up
* Bench Press with Dumbbells
* Butterfly

Shoulder Exercises:
* Standing Shoulder Press
* Seated Shoulder Press
* Lateral Raise
* Front Raise
* Arnold Press
* Upright Row

Strength Exercises (continued)

Leg Exercises:
* Squat
* Sumo Squat
* Bulgarian Squat
* One Legged Deadlift
* Lying Leg Abductors
* Lying Leg Adductors

Calf Exercises:
* Calf Raises
* Dumbbell Calf Raises
* Single Leg Calf Raises

These strength exercises can be done anywhere with only a set of dumbbells or just using your body weight. There is one exercise, hyperextension, that uses an exercise ball, but you could also do it on the floor with a stack of pillows if necessary.

I am confident these exercises will give you a great starting point and allow room for progression. As you learn more exercises and what body parts they work, you can keep adding to the list. This will allow you to keep creating new and different workouts for yourself.

If you do have a gym membership, do not be afraid of the free weights and machines. Incorporating them into your workout can be very beneficial. Most machines have images on them to show you the body part being worked and instructions on how to use it. Also, please do not hesitate to ask someone in the gym for help. I know some of the "gym rats" can seem intimidating, but most are willing to help those who need it. I was one myself, and you never know… you may become one too. Everyone starts as a beginner.

It's Your Turn To Take ACTION!!! Your goal is *strength*! Here are templates to help you create different workouts that you will be able to insert into your weekly routine.

1. Look at the templates.

2. Fill in an exercise from the list above in the template for the appropriate body part.

3. Make sure to select different exercises for each slot.

Strength Workout 1
Chest/ Tricep

Body Part	Exercise for the body part	Sets	Time or Reps	Rest (seconds)
Warm Up	Stretch the chest and tricep muscles	1	5 min	60
Cardio Insert	Jumping Jacks or High Knees	1	100 rep	60
Chest		3	10, 8, 6 rep	60
Chest		3	10, 8, 6 rep	60
Chest		3	10, 8, 6 rep	60
Tricep		3	10, 8, 6 rep	60
Tricep		3	10, 8, 6 rep	60
Tricep		3	10, 8, 6 rep	60
Cardio Insert	Jumping Jacks or High Knees	1	100 rep	60
Cool Down	Stretch the chest and tricep muscles	1	5 min	60

A lot of times when we are ready to hit the weights, we don't think about warming up and stretching;

however, it is important to take that time to warm the muscles and stretch. Warming up your body helps your muscles prepare for lifting. In this case, you want to stretch and loosen the muscles you will be working on specific days.

You may also be wondering why I do not have cardio listed. Jumping jacks and high knees are considered cardio, because it raises the heart rate. You can do other things like jump roping, lateral jumps, squat jumps, jump lunges, burpees, or anything that gets the whole body warm in a short amount of time. This quick cardio assists in getting the body warmed up for resistance training.

I refrain from suggesting long endurance cardio when the goal is building strength. Long endurance cardio is counterproductive, because it will burn up your muscle, which is the opposite of what you want to do when trying to build strength. If you really want to incorporate some cardio into your routine, I would suggest only once a week for no longer than 30 minutes.

You build muscle by tearing up muscle fibers through resistance training and then letting them recover and rebuild those fibers stronger. Recovery of a muscle can take 5-7 days depending on the intensity of the workout, so it is important to give the muscles the rest that they need. Strength workouts may not be fast circuits, but the intensity is still there when you challenge yourself with heavier weights. And you do want to keep challenging yourself with those weights!

Great job in creating your first workout! Let's get started on Workout 2

Strength Workout 2
Back/ Bicep

Body Part	Exercise for the body part	Sets	Time or Rep	Rest (seconds)
Warm Up	Stretch the back and bicep muscles	1	5 min	60
Cardio Insert	Jumping Jacks or High Knees	1	100 rep	60
Back		3	10, 8, 6 rep	60
Back		3	10, 8, 6 rep	60
Back		3	10, 8, 6 rep	60
Bicep		3	10, 8, 6 rep	60
Bicep		3	10, 8, 6 rep	60
Bicep		3	10, 8, 6 rep	60
Cardio Insert	Jumping Jacks or High Knees	1	100 rep	60
Cool Down	Stretch the back and bicep muscles	1	5 min	60

Grouping of the body parts in a specific way can help with getting the most out of your workout. I group back and bicep together, because a lot of the back exercises include pulling movements, which also ignites the bicep muscle. Same with chest and tricep. Chest exercises involve pushing, which ignites the tricep muscle. Grouping these body parts together maximizes the fatigue and usage of those muscle groups in one day and allows it to get better rest for recovery purposes on the other workout days.

Now if you don't have as many days to work out during the week, you can always group upper body exercises together and lower body exercises together to ensure that each group is getting recovery time before being worked again.

Strength Workout 3
Legs/Shoulders

Body Part	Exercise for the body part	Sets	Time or Rep	Rest (seconds)
Warm Up	Stretch the leg and shoulder muscles	1	5 min	60
Cardio Insert	Jumping Jacks or High Knees	1	100 rep	60
Legs		3	10, 8, 6 rep	60
Legs		3	10, 8, 6 rep	60
Legs		3	10, 8, 6 rep	60
Shoulder		3	10, 8, 6 rep	60
Shoulder		3	10, 8, 6 rep	60
Shoulder		3	10, 8, 6 rep	60
Cardio Insert	Jumping Jacks or High Knees	1	100 rep	60
Cool Down	Stretch the leg and shoulder muscles	1	5 min	60

The purpose of strength training is to increase in strength. Now this does not mean that you are going to go from lifting 5 pounds to 20 pounds in a week. It's possible, but it doesn't always work that way. In order to build strength, it is important to keep pushing yourself.

For example, you want to have a light weight, medium weight, and heavy weight. You want to use the light weight on the first set of 10. Move up to the medium weight on the second set of 8, and then use the heavy weight on the last set of 6. It's okay if you don't make 6 reps. It gives you a way to view your progress. Try it again then next time and see if you can get 1 more rep. Just keep working at it! You'll get there!

This allows you to push your muscles even after they are tired. When you hit 6 with your heavy weight multiple times, then it is time to move up in weight.

You won't be able to reach your full potential if you stay with 5 pound weights and never push yourself. It just won't happen.

One more thing! Women who aim for this goal, enjoy their strong muscles. I know I do! So, if someone questions you about wanting to look like a man or being too "muscly", ignore them! If they are making those comments, then they do not know what it takes to accomplish this goal. I assure you that you will not look like a man. As you progress, you are the judge of how far you want to take your strength! It's your journey! Don't let the opinion of others stop you. Once you hit the strength you are happy with, your new goal will be to maintain that strength.

Strength Workout 4
Abs/Cardio

Body Part	Exercise for the body part	Sets	Time or Rep	Rest (seconds)
Warm Up	Stretch the abs and legs muscles	1	5 min	60
Cardio Insert	Jumping Jacks	1	100 rep	30
Abs		3	50 rep	60
Cardio Insert	High Knees	1	100 rep	30
Abs		3	50 rep	60
Cardio Insert	Heel To Butt Fast Jog In Place	1	100 rep	30
Abs		3	50 rep	60
Cardio Insert	Jumping Jacks	1	100 rep	30
Cool Down	Stretch the leg and shoulder muscles	1	5 min	60

I know you may be dying to do some cardio, so here is a way you can incorporate it and not ruin your hard work of strength building.

Ab workouts should focus on feeling the burn. You want that thin and sculpted look for your abs. That is one area that you do not want to be bulkier, so it is not necessary to use heavy weights when working your abs.

During your ab sets, focus on contracting your abs, exhaling on the contraction, and utilizing the rest time to recover for the next set. The cardio portions are high intensity, quick jolts to get the metabolism going. You can add this into the end of your weekly routine if you have time.

Full Body Workouts are NOT as effective in building strength, because working the whole body, every day, doesn't allow time for the muscles to recover and build. Yes, you keep tearing them down, but never give them time to recover and rebuild stronger. This is why for strength building, you are learning how to create body part split workouts. Maximize your workout for the greatest effect!

Ways You Can Adjust These Workouts:

1. If you are limited in dumbbells there are other ways to increase strength that you can try. Negative movements are helpful when building strength. A negative movement is when you quickly contract the muscle and then very slowly release it back to the starting position.

2. To test your strength and keep progressing you can lower the rest time to 15 seconds and do all 3 exercises with that heavy weight. You should not be able to reach 10 reps by the end of the 3rd set. If you do, then you need to move up in weight. This is a good tip to try on the bench press.

3. If you want more muscular endurance and toning, then change the repetitions to 20, 15, 10.

4. If you want to increase your strength even more, then increase the weights and do 6, 4, 2 repetitions. This is for people who are aiming to build extreme muscle and strength.

Once you start building strength and get a feel of the direction you want to go, whether it's more toning or more muscle building, you just adjust the repetitions accordingly and keep aiming for your goal.

Congratulations! You just wrote yourself a workout routine that will help you build strength! You can now work out with a purpose and a goal in mind, rather than random body parts and exercises, hoping to get stronger! WAY TO GO! I can't wait for you to put this to action in the next chapter. When you are ready, You can head on over to **Chapter 10!**

That is where the real fun will begin!

Agility Exercises

Lower Body:
* Tripling High Knees
* Lateral In-In, Out-Out
* Box Jumps
* Tripling Heel To Butt
* Forward Bunny Hop

Full Body:
* Hurdling
* Walk on Balance Beam
* Burpee
* Squat Jumps

Upper Body:
* Ali Shuffle Punch- LOWER BODY, UPPER BODY
* Push-up Clap Incline
* Medicine Ball Chest Throw
* Medicine Ball Hip Throw

Agility requires speed and explosiveness. Focusing on those things through these exercises will help you progress towards your goals. I encourage you NOT to go through the motions if agility is your goal. Focus on executing and exploding in each of these exercises. Practice your speed. Practice, Practice, Practice. You may start off slow, but that's okay. As long as you practice and give it your all, you will keep getting faster. Also, because of the stress put on your body and joints, it is very important to take the time to stretch before and after your workout.

81

It's Your Turn To Take ACTION!!! Your goal is **agility**! Here is a template to help you create different workouts that you will be able to insert into your weekly routine.

1. Look at the template.

2. Pick an exercise from the list above that pertains to your specific agility goals. Whether it be more lower body agility, or incorporating some upper body as well. Just keep switching out exercises to form new workouts.

Agility Workout

Body Part	Exercise for the body part	Sets	Time or Rep	Rest (seconds)
Warm Up	Dynamic stretching	1	5 min	60
Upper Body		5	5 rep	15-30
Lower Body		5	5 rep	15-30
Full Body		5	5 rep	15-30
Upper Body		5	5 rep	15-30
Lower Body		5	5 rep	15-30
Full Body		5	5 rep	15-30
Cool Down	Static Stretch	1	5 min	60

Dynamic Stretching is stretching in a way where you are swinging and moving your joints and ligaments to stretch them out. You can do 10 leg swings forward and backward, 10 Leg swings from side to side, and 10 air squats to warm up. You want to move those joints and get them warm and prepared for speed and explosion.

A Static Stretch is where you press and hold a movement for a period of time. Static stretching would be better at the end of your workout for this goal.

You may notice that I only have 1 workout option for this category. Remember for agility you want to focus on speed in all areas. You want to be well rounded with your performance. So, you can use this same template 3 times a week and insert different exercises for each day. However, agility really focuses on performance and you want to track your progress in how you are performing each exercise, so it is okay to stick to 1 or 2 workouts and do them over and practice those movements to get faster.

Ways You Can Adjust These Workouts:

1. Time yourself. Have a family member count. How long does it take you to do an exercise? Try to improve your time.

2. Add higher level of agility exercises to your workout routine.

Congratulations! You just wrote yourself an agility workout routine, according to YOU! You can now workout with a purpose and a goal in mind, rather than randomly inserting quick movements hoping to be faster and more agile. WAY TO GO! I can't wait for you to put this to action in the next chapter. When you are ready, You can head on over to **Chapter 10!**

That is where the real fun will begin!

Cardiovascular Exercises

* Marching In Place
* Jumping Jacks
* Walking
* Running
* Cycling
* Jump Roping
* Spinning
* Swimming
* Yoga
* Pilates
* Zumba Class
* Any Cardio Machine in the Gym

Cardiovascular Health focuses on endurance and being able to perform an activity for a longer period of time. If you get out of breath easily, then you should be incorporating cardiovascular exercises into your routine. If you need to perform a cardio activity for a very long time, like running in a marathon, then you should be working on cardiovascular exercises. Cardio is an all around great exercise to help build endurance and improve heart health. There are a lot of cardiovascular options out there besides walking and jogging.

It's Your Turn To Take ACTION!!! Your goal is *cardiovascular health*! Here are templates to help you create different workouts that you will be able to insert into your weekly routine and improve your cardiovascular health.

1. Look at the templates.

2. Pick an exercise from the list above and insert them into the templates.

Cardio Workout 1
Level 1

Body Part	Exercise	Sets	Time	Rest (seconds)
Warm Up	Dynamic stretching	1	5 min	60
Cardio		1	10 min	90
Cardio		1	10 min	90
Cardio		1	10 min	90
Cool Down	Static Stretch	1	5 min	60

In this cardio workout, you are building up to 30 minutes of exercise but incorporating multiple cardio exercises. So many people dislike the idea of cardio, because they limit themselves to thinking that it involves walking, running, or the treadmill. Switching up the cardio activity at the beginning of your journey will allow you to have success in increasing that endurance rather than doing the same old exercise for longer periods of time. That just gets boring. Don't be afraid to make cardio fun and enjoyable!

Cardio Workout 2
Level 2

Body Part	Exercise	Sets	Time	Rest (seconds)
Warm Up	Dynamic stretching	1	5 min	60
Cardio		1	25 min	90
Cardio		1	25 min	90
Cool Down	Static Stretch	1	5 min	60

Ultimately your goal is to be able to do one of the cardio exercises for a long period of time. As you improve in your endurance, you may want to get more specific with your exercise choices. If you are training for a bicycle race, you will want to practice spinning and biking. If you are running a marathon, you will want to practice walking, jogging, and eventually running. If you are training for a triathlon, you want to practice swimming, biking, and running. It is optimal to actually train doing the activity that you have to do for the specific event you are participating in. However; you may simply just want to be able to walk up a steep hill, keep up with your kids or grandkids, or walk around the block. Those types of goals allow for more variety in your routine. But the goal is still the same: to increase the time you are able to do those activities. So if you do have more flexibility in your cardio activity, select ones that you enjoy most and insert them into the level 2 workout.

Cardio Workout 3
Level 3

Body Part	Exercise	Sets	Time	Rest (seconds)
Warm Up	Dynamic stretching	1	5 min	60
Cardio		1	60 min	90
Cool Down	Static Stretch	1	5 min	60

I would not incorporate all of these workouts into one week time. You need to get a good feel of how long you can perform cardio comfortably and make the proper adjustments to your time. That is why I have them labeled as level 1, 2, and 3. Start with level 1 until that becomes pretty easy for you. You will feel yourself getting stronger and improving. You will feel the cardio getting easier and you will be able to increase your time by a few minutes. Always strive to increase your time, but remember to stay safe. It is okay to keep the timing the same until you feel yourself getting stronger. Listen to your body! Move to the next level when you feel ready! Remember this is your body and your journey!

Ways You Can Adjust These Workouts:

1. Increase the time that you do each cardio exercise.

2. Either add or take away exercises. Add in a different cardio exercise if you're struggling to stay motivated.

3. You can either set a time goal for the workouts or a mileage goal for the workouts. You would switch out the time slot for a mileage if that is your goal. Whichever you choose, stick to that throughout your routines, so you can track your progress.

4. Once you have improved your cardiovascular health, you can slowly increase the pace in which you perform the activities.

Congratulations! You just wrote yourself a cardiovascular workout routine, according to YOU! You can now workout with a purpose and a goal in mind, rather than randomly walking when you feel like it! WAY TO GO! I can't wait for you to put this to action in the next chapter. When you are ready, You can head on over to **Chapter 10!**

That is where the real fun will begin!

Weight-Loss Exercises

Bicep Exercises:
* Alternating Bicep Curls
* Concentration Curls
* Alternating Hammer Curls
* Seated Double Bicep Curls
* Seated Double Hammer Curls

Tricep Exercises:
* Tricep Dip With Legs Extended
* Close Push-Ups
* Close Push-Ups On Knees
* Seated Tricep Extension
* Chair Dips With Bent Legs
* Chair Dips With Legs Elevated
* Tricep Kickbacks

Back Exercises:
* Superman- LOWER BACK, GLUTES, SHOULDERS
* Reverse Fly- UPPER BACK
* Bent Over Rows- UPPER BACK
* Reverse Grip Bent Over Rows- BACK
* Bird Dog Alternating- BACK, ABS
* Hyperextension Using Exercise Ball- LOWER BACK
* Plank- BACK, ABS, CHEST

Weight-Loss Exercises (continued)

Chest Exercises:
* Push-Up
* Push-Up On Knees
* Wide Push-Up
* Decline Push-Up
* Incline Push-Up
* Bench Press with Dumbbells
* Butterfly

Shoulder Exercises:
* Standing Shoulder Press
* Seated Shoulder Press
* Lateral Raise
* Front Raise
* Arnold Press
* Upright Row

Legs Exercises:
* Squat
* Sumo Squat
* Bulgarian Squat
* One Legged Deadlift
* Lying Leg Abductors
* Lying Leg Adductors

Calf Exercises:
* Calf Raises
* Dumbbell Calf Raises
* Single Leg Calf Raises

Weight-Loss Exercises (continued)

Abdominal Exercises:
* Oblique Crunch- OBLIQUES
* Russian Twist- OBLIQUES
* Bicycle Crunch- OBLIQUES
* Double Crunch- ALL ABS
* Lying Toe Touch- ALL ABS
* Reverse Crunch- LOWER ABS
* Lying Leg Raises- LOWER ABS

Cardio/Full Body Exercises:
* Marching In Place- CARDIO, FULL BODY
* Jumping Jacks- CARDIO, FULL BODY
* Box Jumps- FULL BODY
* Tripling High Knees- FULL BODY
* Walking- CARDIO, LEGS
* Running- CARDIO, LEGS, FULL BODY
* Cycling- CARDIO, LEGS
* Jump Roping- CARDIO, CALVES, FULL BODY
* Spinning- CARDIO, LEGS
* Swimming- CARDIO, FULL BODY
* Any Cardio Machine in the Gym- FULL BODY

Weight-loss exercises can be a combination of strength training exercises and cardio exercises. Combining these two types of exercises in a fast pace workout will burn more calories and help you tone while you lose weight. There are quite a few ways that you can mix up exercises in order to get that higher intensity workout without killing yourself with 100 reps. Circuits, Giant Sets, Supersets, and Intervals are all ways to create weight-loss workouts into your routine. It's also good to rotate through these different ideas to keep things different and new. I also encourage you to find new exercises to keep adding to your list. Check out my website, KatydidFitness.com for more exercise ideas that are also organized by body parts. As you get a good routine in place, it may be something that you will be interested in the future as your journey progresses.

It's Your Turn To Take ACTION!!! Your goal is *weight-loss*! Here are some different templates you can use to help you create different workouts that you will be able to insert into your weekly routine.

1. Look at the templates.

2. Pick an exercise from the list above and insert it into the template.

Weight-loss Workout 1
Full Body Circuit Option

Body Part	Exercise	Sets	Time/ Reps	Rest (second)
Warm Up	Stretch your full body through flexibility moves	1	5 min	60
Chest		1	10 Reps	0
Back		1	10 Reps	0
Tricep		1	10 Reps	0
Bicep		1	10 Reps	0
Shoulder		1	10 Reps	0
Legs		1	10 Reps	0
Calves		1	10 Reps	0
Abs		1	20 Reps	90
	REPEAT LIST AGAIN			
	REPEAT LIST A 3rd TIME			
Cardio		1	20 min intervals or incline	90
Cool Down	Static Stretch	1	5 min	60

A circuit is when you perform a list of 5-8 exercises with little to no rest in between. When doing a circuit, you want to make sure you are going at a quick pace, while keeping your exercise form correct, and you don't stop moving until the circuit is complete. Then rest and do it again. I recommend that you at least do a circuit 2 times. Depending on the time you have available, you can do the circuit 3 or more times, but remember that you want to incorporate a 20 minute interval cardio session as well. I have found that intervals have been very effective in weight-loss. You can choose any activity, but make sure to increase the intensity for 1 minute followed by 2 minutes slow for recovery time.

You are off to a great start in learning how to create your own workouts. Let's check out workout 2.

Weight-loss Workout 2
Giant Set Option

Body Part	Exercise	Sets	Time/ Reps	Rest (seconds)
Warm Up	Stretch your full body through flexibility moves	1	5 min	60
Legs		1	10 reps	0
Shoulder		1	10 reps	0
Abs		1	20 reps	60
	REST Do Giant Set 1 or 2 more times			
Legs		1	10 reps	0
Shoulder		1	10 reps	0
Abs		1	20 reps	60
	REST Do Giant Set 1 or 2 more times			
Legs		1	10 reps	0
Shoulder		1	10 reps	0
Abs		1	20 reps	60
	REST Do Giant Set 1 or 2 more times			
Cardio		1	20 min intervals or incline	90
Cool Down	Static Stretch	1	5 min	60

Giant Sets are usually groups of 3 exercises, but it allows you to focus on specific muscle groups. For example, you can group together *legs/shoulders/abs* in one giant set workout. You could create another giant set workout with the same template using Upper Body: *Chest/Back/Arms* or Lower Body: *Quads/ Glues/Hamstrings.* But like circuits, you do not want to rest until you are done with the giant set. Make sure to pick different exercises for each of the giant sets, because you are doing each giant set 2-3 times total. By the time you're done with your workout, those muscle groups will be totally worked in all different ways!

If you do decide to incorporate giant sets, make sure you give the muscles that you worked time to recover. You can create giant sets for the other body parts as well as taking rest days in order to recover before doing another high intensity workout for that muscle group.

Weight-loss Workout 3
Superset Option

Body Part	Exercise	Set	Time Or Reps	Rest (seconds)
Warm Up	Stretch your full body through flexibility moves	1	5 min	60
Chest		1	10 reps	0
Tricep		1	10 reps	60
	REST Do Superset 2 more times			
Chest		1	10 reps	0
Tricep		1	10 reps	60
	REST Do Superset 2 more times			
Chest		1	10 reps	0
Tricep		1	10 reps	60
	REST Do Superset 2 more times			
Cardio		1	20 min intervals or incline	90
Cool Down	Static Stretch	1	5 min	60

With the Superset option, you can be even more specific with your workouts if you are looking to sculpt and tone as you lose. You can use this template for *chest and tricep*, as well as, *back and bicep*. I group chest and tricep together, because when doing each of these types of exercises you are using a pushing motion which fires both the chest and tricep muscles. Same goes along with back and bicep. Those exercises involve pulling motions which use both muscles groups. Grouping your workout this way allows you to work those muscle groups to the best of their ability and allows for them to recover as you work different areas throughout the week.

Weight-loss Workout 4
Cardio Option

Body Part	Exercise	Set	Time Or Reps	Rest (seconds)
Warm Up	Stretch your full body through flexibility moves	1	5 min	60
Full Body		2	60 sec	60
Full Body		2	60 sec	60
Full Body		2	60 sec	60
Cardio		1	20 min intervals or incline	90
Cool Down	Static Stretch	1	5 min	60

Cardio for weight-loss looks different than cardio for cardiovascular health. It takes more energy to stop and start yourself during a cardio activity than it does to start and keep on going at a constant pace. Think about driving a car. Pressing the gas and brake continuously will burn up more gasoline than just driving at a steady pace. That is the goal with a cardio weight-loss workout. Insert quick cardio exercises like jumping rope, jumping jacks, marching quickly in place, or high knees. I guarantee you'll be sweaty and out of breath.

Ways You Can Adjust These Workouts:

1. With any of these workout options, you can always increase the repetitions. A good range is between 10-20 repetitions. Abs you can do more.

2. You can lengthen your rest time to catch your breath, so you can give your circuits, giant sets, and supersets your all.

3. You can shorten your rest time if you feel that the allotted time is too long.

4. You can change up the intervals by figuring out a comfortable fast and slow time for yourself. You can also decrease the fast and slow times to get more intense.

5. Keep switching out different exercises into the workout templates.

Congratulations! You just wrote yourself a weight-loss workout routine, according to YOU! You can now work out with a purpose and a goal in mind! WAY TO GO! I can't wait for you to put this to action in the next chapter. When you are ready, You can head on over to **Chapter 10!**

That is where the real fun will begin!

Low Impact Exercises for Joint-Health

Chest Exercises:
* Kneeling Thoracic Rotation
* Chest Stretch Standing
* Floor Chest Stretch
* Push-Up On Knees
* Bench Press with Dumbbells
* Butterfly

Tricep Exercises:
* Tricep Stretch Behind Back
* Single Arm Tricep Stretch
* Close Push-Ups On Knees
* Seated Tricep Extension
* Chair Dips With Bent Legs
* Tricep Kickbacks

Bicep Exercises:
* Bicep Stretch Standing
* Alternating Bicep Curls
* Alternating Hammer Curls
* Seated Double Bicep Curls
* Seated Double Hammer Curls

Low Impact Exercises for
Joint-Health (continued)

Back Exercises:
* W-Pump- UPPER BACK, SHOULDERS
* Eagle Supine- LOWER BACK
* Neck Stretch Sideways- NECK
* Windmill-BACK, SHOULDERS
* Bird Dog Alternating- BACK, ABS
* Hyperextension Using Exercise Ball- LOWER BACK

Shoulder Exercises:
* Standing Shoulder Press
* Seated Shoulder Press
* Lateral Raise
* Front Raise
* Upright Row

Leg Exercises:
* Ball Squat
* Ball Sumo Squat
* Lying Leg Abductors
* Lying Leg Adductors
* Leg Extensions On Hands And Knees
* Ankle Mobilization Seated- LEG, FOOT
* Heel To Toe- ANKLE, CALVES
* Leg Swings Front and Back- GLUTES, LEGS
* Leg Swing Sideways
* Bent Over Toe Touch

Low Impact Exercises for Joint-Health (continued)

Calf Exercises:
* Calf Raises
* Single Leg Calf Raises

Abdominal Exercises:
* Rotating Lower Body- ABS
* Bent Leg Core Rotation Lying- OBLIQUES
* Single Leg Dynamic Stretch- ABS, GLUTES
* Oblique Crunch- OBLIQUES
* Russian Twist- OBLIQUES
* Bicycle Crunch- OBLIQUES
* Double Crunch- ALL ABS
* Lying Toe Touch- ALL ABS
* Reverse Crunch- LOWER ABS

Low Impact Cardio Exercises:
* Swimming
* Yoga
* Walking
* Bicycle
* Individual Stepper
* Elliptical
* Water Aerobics

Having the goal of joint-health does not mean that you are stuck in the realm of stretches. There are a lot of options when it comes to low-impact exercises. You just need to know where to begin. Yes, when it comes to your joints, it is important to start very basic in order to avoid injury and strengthen the tendons and ligaments around your joints, but as they get stronger, you will be able to do more.

Know your body. Know your limits. If something hurts, stop and look for an easier exercise that you can do. I've provided a lot of options to choose from specifically for that purpose. Everyone is different, and everyone has different limitations. That's why it's good to keep adding exercises that you can do to your list, so you know what works for you and you can insert them into the templates I provide.

If your condition is more serious, I advise you to consult your doctor first, before starting any exercising. A lot of times your doctor will have safe exercises for you to start with if you are limited in any way. Start there if that is your option. But if you are cleared to exercise, then you can continue with these templates.

It's Your Turn To Take ACTION!!! Your goal is *joint-health*! Here are templates to help you create different workouts that you will be able to insert into your weekly routine.

1. Look at the templates.

2. Fill in an exercise from the list above in the template for the appropriate body part.

3. Make sure to select different exercises for each slot.

Low-Impact Workout 1
Full Body

Body Part	Exercise	Sets	Time Or Reps	Rest (seconds)
Warm Up	Stretch your full body	1	5 min	60
Chest		3	10 Reps	30-60
Back		3	10 Reps	30-60
Tricep		3	10 Reps	30-60
Bicep		3	10 Reps	30-60
Shoulder		3	10 Reps	30-60
Legs		3	10 Reps	30-60
Calves		3	10 Reps	30-60
Abs		3	20 Reps	30-60
Cardio		1	10 min constant pace	90
Cool Down	Static Stretch	1	5 min	60

I recommend full body workouts. Full body workouts are great for moving all the joints in your whole body. Moving your joints allows the synovial fluid to lubricate the joint, helping you to move easier.

If you find that you have swollen joints due to arthritis, regular movement of those joints can help reduce fluid buildup in the joints and will relieve some pain and pressure. So rather than focusing on individual body parts, it is important to have an overall workout that will help benefit the whole body.

With the full body template above, you can create 3 or 4 different workouts just by switching out the exercises for each part.

Low-Impact Workout 2
Cardio

Body Part	Exercise	Sets	Time Or Reps	Rest (seconds)
Warm Up	Stretch your full body	1	5 min	60
Upper Body Mobility		3	10 Reps	30-60
Lower Body Mobility		3	10 Reps	30-60
Cardio		1	20 min Constant pace	60
Cool Down	Static Stretch	1	5 min	60

You can also incorporate a low impact cardio option into your week. I would insert this at least once a week, but make sure to incorporate a full body workout as well to help you build up your strength.

Remember, this is not a high intensity workout. You are not working out for speed and muscle building. These workouts are designed to focus on joint health, stability, and mobilization in a low impact way. Like all workouts, as things get easier and you get stronger, you can increase the level of difficulty with the exercises. But remember, be patient with yourself.

The more you incorporate these workouts, the stronger you will get.

Ways You Can Adjust These Workouts:

1. Give yourself more rest if you need more rest, but utilize the windows of time in which you are feeling good to keep moving.

2. Switch out the exercises often to create a new workout and keep the body moving.

3. Keep the resistance low until you feel like the movements are getting easy for you.

4. You can start increasing resistance if you feel like you are getting stronger.

Congratulations! You just wrote yourself a joint-health workout routine, according to YOU! You can now work out with a purpose and a goal in mind! WAY TO GO! I can't wait for you to put this to action in the next chapter. When you are ready, You can head on over to **Chapter 10!**

That is where the real fun will begin!

Chapter 10

YOUR FITNESS CHALLENGE

We are what we repeatedly do. Excellence, therefore, is not an act but a habit." -Aristotle.

You are amazing! Do you know how far you've come? You have all the tools to be successful throughout your journey! That is exciting! Now it's time to put it all into action!

Throughout this book, I have provided you with ways to help you encourage yourself when others won't. You have figured out the WHY for even starting this journey. You have determined your goal, organized your schedule, and created goal oriented workouts just for YOU! That is AMAZING!!! If you have followed all of my instructions so far, you have begun building a solid foundation for long term results!

See, everything that I have discussed previously is what a lot of women rush through, because they want to get right into working out for quick results. What they don't realize is, that if they do not really get a grasp of how to actually incorporate the workouts and build the foundation of making it a lifestyle, then they

113

will do the workouts for a while, but then get bored or worse....appear to reach their goal, then be happy that they accomplished something and go right back to their old, unhealthy path.

If you skipped any of the previous chapters, I strongly urge you to go back and really reflect and put into action the topics and ideas that I discuss to build that foundation. It's not all rainbows and butterflies. It will get tiring. It will get boring. It will get tedious, but the foundation and positive self-talk will help you through it. And as it becomes habit and a lifestyle, then it won't feel boring and tedious anymore. It will become as much of your daily or weekly routine as showering.

Okay, enough chit chat. Let's get this challenge started! I challenge you to incorporate everything you've learned for the next 28 days!

On the following pages you will have to readdress your WHY, some positive self-talk phrases that work for you, your goal, the days that work best for you and the time frame in which you have time to workout. Don't just guess. You did figure this all out in previous chapters, so go back and look at what you wrote.

This is your journey. This is all based on you! No short cuts. It will all be worth it in the long run, trust me. You have come this far. You can keep on going! Remember, you are stronger than you think. You can endure more than you think. You do have the power to change your habits. And most of all, YOU ARE WORTH IT! You can do this!

My 28 Day Challenge

Positive Self-Talk Phrases That Work For Me:

1. _____

2. _____

3. _____

4. _____

My WHY:

My Goal:

I am using the _____ Exercise Templates.

Before You Begin

My Beginning Weight is: _____

A healthy weight-loss is 1-2 lbs a week. Some lose more and some lose less depending on how far along in their journey they are, but if you see that you are only losing 1-2 lbs per week, I reassure you that this is totally normal and you are losing at a pace in which your body can adjust and keep up with your weight-loss.

115

Also, it is possible to be up to 4 lbs heavier at the end of the day, just by the food and liquids you drink throughout that day. So, if you are someone who just weighs yourself randomly, you might find yourself quite frustrated and not seeing progress like you had hoped. My recommendation is to weigh and measure yourself first thing in the morning before you eat breakfast and be consistent with the time in which you measure throughout the 30 days in order to get the most accurate readings. And do not keep weighing yourself throughout the day…that will kill your spirit!

Before Photos: Make sure to take them and keep them somewhere where you will be able to compare.

When taking your progress photos, you want to make sure to wear something that is tight or somewhat revealing like a sports bra and leggings/shorts. If you wear something baggy and loose, you will not be able to see all the progress you've made.   Also, make sure to wear the same outfit, or something similar, for all progress pictures if possible. This will allow you to see true progress rather than changes seen from wearing tighter pants. Take a Front, Side, and Back shot of yourself.

Measurements: Record in centimeters or inches, but keep it consistent throughout the 28 days.

Chest (over the bust)	
Right Arm	
Left Arm	
Waist (across belly button)	
Hips	
Right Thigh	
Left Thigh	
	Total:

WEEK 1

This Week: These Days of the Week Generally Work Best For Me: (circle at least 3 of them) MONDAY. TUESDAY, WEDNESDAY, THURSDAY, FRIDAY, SATURDAY, SUNDAY

Check off the day once you complete a workout.

☐ **Sunday:** Time of Workout: _____
Description of workout: _____

☐ **Monday:** Time of Workout: _____
Description of workout: _____

☐ **Tuesday:** Time of Workout: _____

Description of workout: _____

☐ **Wednesday:** Time of Workout: _____

Description of workout: _____

☐ **Thursday:** Time of Workout: _____

Description of workout: _____

☐ **Friday:** Time of Workout: _____

Description of workout: _____

☐ **Saturday:** Time of Workout: _____

Description of workout: _____

You Competed Week 1! You're a Rock Star! Keep Going!

WEEK 2

This Week: These Days of the Week Generally Work Best For Me: (circle at least 3 of them) MONDAY. TUESDAY, WEDNESDAY, THURSDAY, FRIDAY, SATURDAY, SUNDAY

Record Weight and Measurements. Check off the day once you complete a workout.

My Weight: _____

Chest	
Right Arm	
Left Arm	
Waist	
Hips	
Right Thigh	
Left Thigh	
	Total:

Pounds/Kilograms Lost (between 1st and 2nd weigh in): _____

Inches/Centimeters Lost (between 1st and 2nd measurements): _____

☐ **Sunday:** Time of Workout: _____

Description of workout: _____

☐ **Monday:** Time of Workout: _____

Description of workout: _____

☐ **Tuesday:** Time of Workout: _____

Description of workout: _____

☐ **Wednesday:** Time of Workout: _____

Description of workout: _____

☐ **Thursday:** Time of Workout: _____

Description of workout: _____

☐ **Friday:** Time of Workout: _____

Description of workout: _____

☐ **Saturday:** Time of Workout: _____

Description of workout: _____

Two weeks down! Awesome work! You are stronger than you were last week. I'm sure this week was tough, but you are still running on the adrenaline and excitement of doing this challenge. That's great! But remember that when things start getting hard to refer to your Positive Self-Talk Strategies and keep on going!

It's Time To Reflect: Think about what has been hard for you the last two weeks. Think about what has been easy. Write down some of your struggles and successes to help you narrow down what you might need to focus more on the next two weeks.

Things I struggled with:

Things I rocked at:

Things I will work on improving the next 2 weeks:

My game plan as to how I will improve these things in the upcoming weeks:

WEEK 3

This Week: These Days of the Week Generally Work Best For Me: (circle at least 3 of them) MONDAY. TUESDAY, WEDNESDAY, THURSDAY, FRIDAY, SATURDAY, SUNDAY

Record Weight and Measurements. Check off the day once you complete a workout.

My Weight is: _____

Chest	
Right Arm	
Left Arm	
Waist	
Hips	
Right Thigh	
Left Thigh	
	Total:

Pounds/Kilograms Lost (between 1st and 3rd weigh-in): _____

Inches/Centimeters Lost (between 1st and 3rd measurements): _____

☐ **Sunday:** Time of Workout: _____
Description of workout: _____

☐ **Monday:** Time of Workout: _____
Description of workout: _____

☐ **Tuesday:** Time of Workout: _____
Description of workout: _____

☐ **Wednesday:** Time of Workout: _____
Description of workout: _____

☐ **Thursday:** Time of Workout: _____
Description of workout: _____

☐ **Friday:** Time of Workout: _____
Description of workout: _____

☐ **Saturday:** Time of Workout: _____
Description of workout: _____

Was this a challenging week for you? You may be feeling tired by now. You might be experiencing muscle soreness, because you are working out in a different way than you're used to. This is all normal. I've been right where you are. But this challenge is a challenge for a reason. You started it with the intension of finishing it. You can do this! Look back at your WHY and your goal! See how you've progressed in the last 3 weeks. Don't just look at the numbers. Pay attention to how you are feeling. How do your pants fit? How is your mood? Are you getting stronger, less out of breath, more confident? Those things matter too! And the longer you stick with it, the more you'll see change! You're doing great so far. You have only one week left! Stay strong! You CAN do this!

WEEK 4

This Week: These Days of the Week Generally Work Best For Me: (circle at least 3 of them) MONDAY. TUESDAY, WEDNESDAY, THURSDAY, FRIDAY, SATURDAY, SUNDAY

Record Weight and Measurements. Check off the day once you complete a workout.

My Weight is: _____

Chest	
Right Arm	
Left Arm	
Waist	
Hips	
Right Thigh	
Left Thigh	
	Total:

Pounds/Kilograms Lost (between the 1st and 4th weigh-in)**: _____**

Inches/Centimeters Lost (between the 1st and 4th measurements)**: _____**

☐ **Sunday:** Time of Workout: _____
   Description of workout: _____

☐ **Monday:** Time of Workout: _____
   Description of workout: _____

☐ **Tuesday:** Time of Workout: _____
   Description of workout: _____

☐ **Wednesday:** Time of Workout: _____
   Description of workout: _____

☐ **Thursday:** Time of Workout: _____
   Description of workout: _____

☐ **Friday:** Time of Workout: _____
   Description of workout: _____

☐ **Saturday:** Time of Workout: _____
   Description of workout: _____

YOU DID IT! You completed 28 days of consistency! Now Let's take our final weight, measurements, and photos to see how much you've accomplished.

My Weight is: _____

Final Measurements:

Chest	
Right Arm	
Left Arm	
Waist	
Hips	
Right Thigh	
Left Thigh	
	Total:

Pounds/Kilograms Lost During The Challenge:

_____

Inches/Centimeters Lost During The Challenge:

_____

When it comes to results, many women have different outcomes. Some women might lose more weight than inches. Other women might more inches/cm than weight. Some may see the changes in their photographs and not as much in the numbers. It's important to take notice of the way that you see your changes, because this will probably be the pattern in which you continue to lose as you progress through your journey.

It doesn't matter if one girl loses more weight. It doesn't matter if another girl loses more inches. The important take away from this challenge is to see what YOUR progress is. Figure out how much you've lost. Celebrate your own accomplishments. We are not here to compare ourselves to anyone else except ourselves. We are setting our own personal records here.

Don't Forget To Take Your After Photos!

Are you happy it's over? Make sure to take another set of pictures and place them next to your Before photos. You should be proud of what you accomplished so far, but guess what? You have just begun. I encourage you to use this template and do it again! Keep going until it becomes routine. If you started with only working out one day a week, I challenge you to add a day. The goal is at least three days a week! If you did three days a week, did you feel like it was still a chore to fit the workouts into your schedule? If so, you need to do this challenge again keeping the 3 day workouts. If you felt that this challenge was easy, I challenge you to increase your days to 4! Take it up a notch if you're ready.

You need to do this challenge until you are doing this challenge without thinking. That is the point of all of this. This should be your routine without even thinking. It takes time to get to this point. Be patient with yourself. Keep looking at your WHY. Keep striving for your goal. Keep telling yourself that you will get there, because if you keep trying...you WILL get there!

Every time you complete this challenge you deserve to celebrate. It's another 28 days of trying your best. Each time, you are closer to your goal. You are closer to discovering a healthy you.

Guess what?! If you complete this challenge 3 times, you have created and completed your very own 12 week workout program! You are truly creating your own that fits you and your goals...at your level! That is life changing!

Chapter 11

WHY NUTRITION

"Let food be thy medicine and medicine be thy food."
-Hippocrates

While working as a personal trainer and through my own personal fitness journey, I have found that individuals who only focus on their workouts eventually need to face the facts about their nutrition. I'm guilty!   I'm part Italian and grew up on pasta! Even though it's probably the last thing you want to hear, exercising can only take you so far.   Your nutrition is extremely important and will offer the secrets you need to discover a healthy you.

The proper nutrition, according to your body, will provide you with healthy habits and foods within the right number of calories, along with a healthy balance of nutrients to help your body function and perform at an optimal level and help you achieve the health and fitness goals you have set out to accomplish.

Everyone wants to make nutrition a complicated task. If you want to make it complicated, there are a million ways to do that.   Or you can start basic, create the healthy foundation, and work your way up to more complex strategies as you develop the foundational habits of healthy living, progress, and want to break plateaus that you might face along the way.

You may find yourself saying, "I try to eat healthy." But in reality you may also find yourself snacking and eating frequent desserts throughout the day. You may say, "I hate tracking my food." But if you want to make an improvement, it is important to keep track of what is working and what is not working. There are many levels of tracking, but it is important to track at some level in order to see progress. You may say, "I track my food, but I don't see any changes." Then something needs to be adjusted, and I will help you do that in the upcoming chapters. You may say, "I watch what I eat." But then you may realize that you are eating a lot less than your body actually needs to achieve your goals.

Everyone is different. Every goal is different. Everyone's daily routines are different. Everyone eats different foods. So it is important to realize where you need to start. Similar to exercise, if you get too complex before you're ready, you will become overwhelmed and quit, because you're discouraged and your mindset will become negative. Set yourself up for success, not failure.

In the upcoming chapters, I will reveal that there are a lot more levels of nutrition than you may think: Basic Healthy Habits, Caloric Intake, Macronutrients, and Supplementation. Not everyone has to start at the same level. Figure out where you need to begin and start there. As you read through the upcoming chapters, you'll quickly realize if you already have a good grasp on the level and can move on to something a little more challenging.

It's Time To Reflect!

Do I track my nutrition? YES   NO   I TRY

If yes, how do I track my nutrition? You may think you don't track, but even counting how many times you eat veggies or how many glasses of water is a form of tracking, so count it.

What do I feel I need to work on with my nutrition?

__Chapter 12__

Your Daily Food Habits

"By cleansing your body on a regular basis and eliminating as many toxins as possible from your environment, your body can begin to heal itself, prevent disease, and become stronger and more resilient than you ever dreamed possible!"
~Dr. Edward Group III

Now that we understand that nutrition doesn't have to be complicated and there are many levels, we are going to start with the basics. It is important to know where you are coming from in order to know where you are headed. So this chapter is not only going to help you discover your current eating habits, but help you figure out where and how you should tweak some of these practical nutrition habits.

Before we get started, I know you are dreading this and probably reluctant to even fill in the reflection section of this chapter, but I promise you that if you just take one question at a time and are honest with yourself you will be a whole lot clearer on what you need to work on in your personal journey. So many times we look at what everyone else is doing and the extreme fad diets out there and want to hop on the band wagon, but this isn't about what is popular. This is about what is right for you and appropriate for you. So take a deep breath, and just take one question at a time.

It's Time To Reflect! Answer the questions honestly. It's okay to be scared. But it's important to work past that fear and keep on stepping and working towards your goals.

How many meals do I eat in a day?

How many times a week do I eat out?

How many frozen meals (pre-made meals) **do I eat per week?**

How many oz of soda/pop do I drink in a day?

How many oz of water do I drink in a day?

How many alcoholic beverages do I drink a week?

Do I crave salty snacks or sweet snacks?

Do I like vegetables?

How many times a day do I eat vegetables?

Which veggies do I like to eat?

Which veggies DON'T I like to eat?

Do I like fruit?

How many times a day do I eat fruit?

Which fruits do I like to eat?

Which fruits DON'T I like to eat?

Do I like starchy carbohydrates (bread, bagels, rice, potatoes, cereals, granola bars)**?**

How many times a day do I eat starchy carbs?

Which starchy carbs do I like to eat?

Which starchy carbs DON'T I like to eat?

Do I like meat/fish?

How many times a day do I eat meat/fish?

Which meats/fish do I like to eat?

Which meats/fish DON'T I like to eat?

Do I like foods that contain healthy fats?
Yes   No   I Don't Know

Which nuts/cheeses/dressings do I like to eat?

I am allergic to these foods:

I get _____ hours sleep each night.

Great work! Congratulations on being completely honest with your habits and likes and dislikes. Below, I will break down each question and provide you with helpful guidance and information based on general possible responses, so you can get a good idea of what you need to work on and how you can tweak your daily routine in a healthier way. Let's get started!

How many meals do I eat in a day?

This topic is highly debatable in the fitness world, but here is the bottom line with being healthy. Getting the correct calorie intake during your day is crucial.

You can eat a few times a day and reach your goals as long as you hit your calorie goals. You can eat 6 times a day and hit your calorie target that is appropriate for your goal. The question you really need to answer is, which one will you be consistent with and hit your calorie target goal as you eat your meals throughout the day?

If you eat too little calories, your body can reach starvation mode and make it difficult to lose weight. If you eat excessively more calories, then you will gain weight. You need to find that sweet spot. And that sweet spot is your calorie range depending on your goal. I will discuss this in more detail in the next

135

chapter.

Another thing to consider when you look at your current eating routine. Your age and metabolism. As you age, your metabolism naturally slows down. Exercise and eating habits have the ability to speed up your metabolism to an extent. Eating, in particular, speeds up your metabolism by processing your food and through absorption. Your body is working to send all the nutrients to the proper locations in your body.

If you only eat 1 meal a day and you are over 35, your metabolism is already starting to slow, and 1 meal a day is not going to speed it up much. But as you eat smaller meals more frequently, your body will start metabolizing those foods as they enter your body. Your body adjusts to the intake and will speed up to distribute the nutrients to where they need to be.

Keep that in mind when you choose your meals throughout the day. I know life is busy, but I would recommend at least 3 meals a day...if not more, especially as we get older. But no matter how many times you eat in a day, remember to make sure you are intaking the proper calories for your goal and are consistent. And if weight-loss is your goal, and calories are confusing to you right now, just remember tweaking some unhealthy habits will decrease your calories automatically and help you see changes in a positive way.

How many times a week do I eat out?

Depending on your fitness goals, determines how many times you can get away with eating out. The leaner you want to be, the less you should eat out. Not that restaurants aren't healthy, but they always have a secret sauce or oils/butters that the food is cooked in, so you really don't know if the nutrition information is correct if they provide any at all. Restaurants have higher amounts of processed foods, just because it needs to last and with processed foods comes a higher sodium count. Sodium makes your body feel bloated and hold water. So if you are looking to lose weight, sodium isn't exactly your friend.

If you are looking to make healthier choices, then I recommend looking at the nutrition menu if it's available and take a look at the calories. A lot of menus now a days offer healthier options. If you are eating out, don't be afraid to ask your server if they could make a substitution for you to make it slightly healthier; however, I wouldn't rely on this. I recommend that you learn what the healthy foods are, so you can determine for yourself what a healthier choice would be.

A lot of times busy women turn to fast food as a quick dinner option because they are just so tired. I get it. It's easy and takes no thought or preparation. But that is not a healthy habit to have. Turning to the lazy way out while you are wanting to stay motivated for your goals is not the answer. That will make you more lazy and less motivated. If you are going to be motivated, try to make all your choices healthier and with intent. I know...easier said than done. But that's why we are working on creating healthier habits, that turn into a lifestyle that you want to have. You don't want to be the mom who goes to the drive thru every day. You don't want to be the mom who throws a donut at their kids for breakfast. Those habits won't help you or your family find a healthy lifestyle. That is pressing the Easy Button and using excuses to make it okay.

So let's start planning more and eating out less. And if you have to eat out, then plan ahead by looking at the nutrition menus, asking for substitutions, or even cutting a portion in half.

Another thing to note. I am not talking about never eating out. I celebrate. I go out to eat. I enjoy special days. One day of eating out does not ruin your goals. It is the continuous habit of eating out that will squash them. So if you find yourself eating out 2 or more times a week (weekends count as part of the week also), then take a look at what you are ordering, the nutrition labels, and see how you can cut back or make those choices healthier. You are strong enough to do this! It just takes doing it.

How many frozen meals (pre-made meals) **do I eat per week?**

Frozen meals you find in the grocery store are the ones pre-made and all ready for you to heat up and eat. In my opinion, these meals are sometimes as bad as eating out. Look at the sodium content on the labels. Look at the calories. Look at the carbohydrates. Look at the saturated fats. If you only have a little bit to lose, the sodium content alone could be stopping you from making progress. The calories are also on the high side, which might put you over your targeted calorie range by the end of the day.

Yes these meals are easy and quick, but the nutritional value isn't as good as fresh or frozen foods with individual ingredients, like chicken and frozen broccoli. Eating out and pre-made frozen meals will slow down your progress, so work on limiting these.

How many ounces of soda/pop do I drink in a day?

The problem that ends up happening with soda/pop, is that it ends up leading to someone drinking most of their calories for the day. This leads to being over on your caloric range and can lead to weight gain. It's also high in carbohydrates/sugar, so if your body type doesn't process carbohydrates very well, then you may be finding that you are not getting anywhere with your weight loss journey. So if you do drink multiple cans/bottles of soda a day, and eat 3 meals a day with it, it is possible you are over doing the intake in calories, which can lead to weight-gain.

The goal is to switch over to water. If this is a struggle for you, it will take time. Be patient with yourself and work on weaning yourself back. The key is to find a healthier replacement for the soda.   I went from drinking Regular Soda multiple times a day, to Diet Soda.   During this time, I was keeping track of my calories and Diet Soda had 0 calories, so that is all I cared about at the time.   I was not aware of the nutrition content and such at the time, and personally didn't care.   All I cared about at the time was my caloric intake and Diet Soda allowed me to still drink it without the calories.

However, I hit a plateau and needed to improve more, so I switched to sparkling water. From the sparkling water, I learned to add fruit and lemon to my ordinary water to make it bearable.   This process that I discussed took me well over a year or maybe even 2 to progress through and work towards, because I wasn't fully ready to commit to going cold turkey.

You might be motivated now, but will you be motivated 10 weeks from now? You need to think about what you can be consistent with and what you can handle long term. I wasn't ready to just drink water and give up my soda, but I could switch to diet. Then when I was there, it was easier for me to find a sparkling water that I enjoyed. What are you ready for? It's okay to go slow. It's okay to jump right in. Figure out what you can be consistent with and what you can work on. Consistency with the healthier choice is the key.

How many ounces of water do I drink in a day?

Water has many benefits. When it comes to your health and fitness journey, water flushes out toxins, boosts energy, helps regulate body temperature, aids in keeping your bowels regular, aids in weight loss, prevents headaches, improves complexion, and prevents cramping in the muscles.

So how much water should you be drinking each day? A simple answer is about 1/2 your body weight in ounces. Depending on your level of exercise, you may want to aim for more.

Before preparing for my figure competition in Las Vegas, I dehydrated on purpose. This is to shed as much water weight as I can, so my muscularity shows through. My situation was a little more complex than what others experience. I do not sweat. It takes me 20 minutes to start sweating on a treadmill when it only takes other people 5 minutes. I need to wear a sweatsuit if I need to shed some serious sweat, so it was quite difficult to shed water and dehydrate. I had to work at it harder and longer. During my dehydration period, I had experienced cramping while trying to flex and hold a pose, the inability to go to the bathroom, headaches, and inability to focus and thing clearly. I sucked on ice chips to get a little water. I was so thirsty after my show, all I wanted to do was drink. I was unaware, that after being so dehydrated that you can actually get water poisoning, which can be fatal. Luckily, I was okay, but I drank so much water, my body literally puffed up. Needless to say I learned my lesson and I never did that again. I eased my body back into a hydrated state and let it adjust.

Dehydration is serious, and you never want to let your body experience it at that level, so it is important to find a way that helps you increase that water intake, so you can enjoy the benefits and not the effects of dehydration. If you ever get to the point where you feel really thirsty, your body is already dehydrated.

I've come across some women who number water bottles. Some pick a favorite water bottle and keep refilling it. Others, like me, fill up a huge jug of water and refill their other glasses of water from that job during the day. Whatever way you choose, once again, consistency is key. Find a way that works for you. Who cares what anyone else is doing? Their

142

way might not work for you. Find a way that works for you and use it daily. Increase that water intake.

How many alcoholic beverages do I drink a week?

This topic can go two ways. You either have to have your glass of wine or alcoholic beverage, or you don't. I can leave it, because my weakness is coffee creamer and chocolate. My husband on the other hand, loves his glass of wine to unwind after work. But is it really helpful in fitness goals to drink a glass of wine every single night? He's tried only having one on his weekends. That didn't last. He's tried going cold turkey. That didn't last either. I found a way in which he could have his glass of wine each night if he really wanted it and still meet his fitness goals.

So what would you have to do in order to have that drink? Well, once again, like the soda, alcohol is sugary carbohydrates and is filled with empty calories. So if you're not careful, drinking alcohol will end up leading you into a surplus of calories that is not in line with your goals. That is what causes weight gain. Not only that, it can throw off your healthy balance of macronutrients that your need for your body to perform at optimal level.

So I personally figured out a balanced plan with foods he regularly eats along with room for a glass of wine. Of course he is trying to cut back to only having a glass on his weekend, but if he fails at that attempt after a long day, as long as he stays within his balanced plan he will be able to enjoy a glass of wine and not go backwards with his goals.

To sum up what I've discussed so far, just simply cutting back on the bad habits will decrease your calories automatically by around 200 calories or even a lot more. So if you've come across one of these topics that is an obstacle in your day, make a small goal for yourself and work on cutting back on one thing until that becomes routine. Then move on to something else.

Every time you work on something new, as long as you are continuing to be consistent and working on the previous task, as well, you will be well on your way to a healthier you!

Do I crave salty snacks or sweet snacks?

CRAVINGS!!! So many women have them. So many women have very little self control when it comes to them. And if you think you have self control, you possibly lose it once a month before and during your cycle. So what is the way around it? I'm just as guilty as everyone else! Chocolate is my sweet weakness.

I started off by watching my intake. I mean, when I had ice cream, I not only had ice cream, but I'd top it with cherries, chocolate syrup, melted peanut butter, and sprinkles. When I had cookies, I wouldn't stop at just 1 or 2. I would eat as many as I could grab in a handful and dip it in milk. Like, I'm serious about my sweets. However, when I started counting my calories figuring out how much I was able to eat to reach my goal, I realized that I was eating way to many sweets and needed to get it under control.

To do this, I simply started by cutting back on portions. Honestly, I couldn't stick with that, because I was someone who would sneak in a few more and maybe not count it in my calories. So, because I knew I didn't have self control, I had to cut it out completely for a while, until I got my calories under control with my other food. When I figured out how to incorporate sweets back in, I began reading labels and looking at the low calorie snack packs. These prepackaged sweets were the perfect treat for me, because I was able to take a whole bag and enjoy everything inside. I'm almost certain it was my mind playing tricks on me and that is what my issue was in the first place. I needed to feel like I wasn't being deprived of it. So eating the individual snack packs helped me enjoy the sweet taste and be okay with being done once I finished the little bag.

Once I did that for a while, I began finding healthier replacements. Let's face it, these snacks might be low calories, but most likely have very little nutrients in it. This is when I discovered little hacks like dark chocolate chips and mixed nuts. A rice cake with Almond Butter and banana slices drizzled with Honey was another one of my favorites.

Now, I am perfectly happy with my cup of coffee and a small portion of dark chocolate chips and cashews as my nighttime snack. After finding the balanced nutrition my body needed, which I did not have in the past, I no longer have any crazy cravings like I used to have earlier in my journey.

Do I like vegetables?

If the answer to this question is yes, then that's wonderful! Vegetables are one of the best things you can start incorporating into your daily nutrition. They are low in calories, low in carbs, but packed full of nutrients which have healing powers for your body.

If your answer is no, then we need to do some brainstorming. If you rarely eat vegetables, you may be deficient in some vitamins and minerals. I would get checked and see if that is the case. If so, then you can start eating the food that has the vitamin or mineral that you are deficient in, or make sure to take that supplement. You can also get a Greens supplement if you are someone that knows that you will not eat your veggies. You don't like them. You don't want to eat them. If this is the case, then they need to be supplemented. You can sprinkle the Greens powder on your food lightly or put it in a smoothy. However you want to take it, but it is important to get it somehow.

How many times a day do I eat vegetables?

Because veggies are the top carbohydrate food that you should be eating, a general rule of thumb is that you should be eating 4 servings of veggies for every 1 serving of fruit. So before you eat that orange or banana, ask yourself how many veggies you had today.

Which veggies do I like to eat?

Write a list of veggies that you love to eat. This will be your go to for your grocery list. Fresh and frozen are great options. If you must do canned, make sure to rinse them first. Corn and carrots are higher in sugar, so I wouldn't make these your go to veggies, but it won't hurt to have them every so often. Green veggies should be priority, but a mixture of all veggies is great! It's better than nothing!

Which veggies DON'T I like to eat?

This list is what you will not pass through those lips. That is okay! You now know what they are. Select different ones! If you don't like veggies at all, then make sure to look into a supplement or ask your doctor what he/she would recommend if there are any deficiencies.

Do I like fruit?

You would think that the answer to this question is a no brainer, but I have come across more people than I actually thought I would that do not eat fruit. So of course this is a legitimate question.

Fruit has slightly higher carbohydrates/sugars and calories than vegetables. So too much fruit is a possibilities, because it can increase your blood sugar levels higher than you want as well as put you over in your calorie range intake if you combine fruit with starchy and sugary carbs. Yes, fruit is healthy for you, but there is such thing as too much of a good thing.

How many times a day do I eat fruit?

Do you remember in the previous section with the vegetables I gave the ratio of 4 veggies to 1 fruit? That is how you can gauge your intake. If you've had a good bit of veggies already, then you can choose a piece of fruit or add some to your protein shake.

Fruits are beneficial. Citrus fruits, kiwi, mango, strawberries, papaya, limes, and lemons all have Vitamin C. Berries contain Vitamin B7 (biotin). Bananas contain vitamin B6. And the list can go on. There are lots of benefits to incorporating fruits into your daily nutrition, so finding that balance is important.

Which fruits do I like to eat?

Make that list of healthy fruits that you like eating. Once again, this will be your go to list when you are creating your grocery list every week. Try to rotate through your choices rather than picking the same ones each time. My kids even enjoy trying out new fruits that none of us have ever tried before. If we don't like it, we know not to get it again. But if we do, then it's one more fruit we can add to our list.

Which fruits DON'T I like to eat?

If you are not a fruit eater, please check with your doctor and get tested for deficiencies. This will tell you what vitamins and minerals you might need to supplement. The real food is best, but if you need to supplement something that your nutrition isn't getting, then that's what you need to do. Your doctor can also help you figure that out as well.

Do I like starchy carbohydrates

Starchy carbohydrates contain higher calories than both veggies and fruits. This is also the most popular category in that it is the one category that gets eaten every meal.

How many times a day do I eat starchy carbs?

Think about it: Toast, Pancakes, Oatmeal, Waffles, Bagels, tortilla wraps, potatoes, rice, pasta, etc. You can find a starchy carbohydrates very easily for every single meal of your day. This is the one category that you can overeat and reverse your progress.

I'm not saying cut these items out completely. No way! Your brain actually needs carbohydrates to function properly. But don't forget that vegetables and fruits are also considered carbohydrates and provide you with nutrients as well.

Look at Quantity and Quality. First of all, if you just cut your portions of your starchy carbs in half of what you are used to eating, you would decrease your calories by a good 300 calories and still be eating starchy carbohydrates. That is enough of a decrease to see progress right off the start. If you did nothing else! Imagine that! Simply cut your toast in half. Eat half serving of rice. Have Half of that bagel. It can all make a huge difference at the end of the day.

When it comes to quality. Not all starchy carbs are created equal. You want to choose non processed, fresh carbohydrates like sweet potatoes, red potatoes, whole wheat products. Avoid the White Flour bread. Choose a bowl of oatmeal over a stack of frozen pancakes. Choose whole wheat bread/buns over white bread/buns. Quality in the ingredients will effect your body on the inside. So combine the quality of your starchy carbohydrate with the quantity adjustment of your starchy carbohydrate and you'll be definitely on the right track to a healthier YOU.

Which starchy carbs do I like to eat?

Make a list of your starchy carbs. Go back to your list and circle it if it is a non processed quality starchy carb. If it is, then great! If not, know that you will really need to look at portions and the label. Or see if there is a whole wheat food similar that you can try instead to replace the unhealthier option.

Which starchy carbs DON'T I like to eat?

Chances are you didn't have a problem writing down ones you like. Unless you have an allergy of some sort. If you can't eat starchy carbohydrates for some reason, this is when you want to increase your vegetable and fruit intake, which is a good thing to do anyways.

I have to stop right here for a moment and applaud you for making it this far! You are making some great realizations about your own habits, likes, and dislikes. This information alone will set you on the right path towards a healthier you. Don't be afraid to go back to your own answers to these questions and add notes next to them to help guide you in your decision making.

Do I like meat/fish?

There is no right or wrong answer to this question. Whether you're a meat lover, vegan, or vegetarian; it is okay. You can still hit your health and fitness goals. The issue comes in when you are not getting enough protein. No matter what kind of foods you eat, the majority of the general population, now a days, are falling short on their protein intake. Meat isn't the only food that contains protein. It just has the highest level of it. That is the issue to be aware of. How many grams of protein are you eating in a day. You should be eating : your body weight in lbs x .8 = g of protein. I am 123 lbs. I should be eating at least 98.4g of protein a day. I aim between .8-1g per body weight. So I aim between 98-123g of protein each day.

Protein is essential in building strong muscles and in your health in general. As you deplete your amino acids in your muscles through exercise and other chores, eating protein will restore that amino acid pool that your body won't naturally produce. You must get it through food. That's why your protein intake is so important. And if you're not reaching your allotted amount for the day, then I recommend that you supplement with a protein shake. They offer a wide variety of shakes out there. I recommend that you find one that is at least 24g of protein. I have found that for those who eat meat, that is a good amount to help assist in reaching your protein goal.

If you do not eat meat, I have found that hemp protein has a high protein content with 11g and you'll want to find other sources of protein through lentils, beans, nuts, tofu, tempeh, seitan, quinoa, and veggie burgers.

How many times a day do I eat meat/fish?

You want to eat protein for every meal of the day. That means at least 3 times a day. You may have it more if you eat snacks throughout your day. Cheeses and nuts also contain protein as well, so don't think that you must eat meat to get a little protein; however, eating those higher protein foods will help you reach your daily protein goal.

Which meats/fish do I like to eat?

Start here with eating the meats and fish you like. Don't be afraid to try new things or prepare them in a different way. Try to avoid breading the meat. If you do, you can use oats instead of bread crumbs. I also like to play with spices when cooking.

Which meats/fish DON'T I like to eat?

Well now you know what you don't like to eat. Try to find something else. If you don't eat meat, look for some foods with higher protein content that isn't meat. It's out there, I promise.

Do I like foods that contain healthy fats?

Healthy fats? What's that?! Are you able to tell the difference between what foods have more saturated and unsaturated fats? Foods like olive oil, avocados, peanuts, pecans, almonds, fish, hemp, flax, and safflower. These are healthy fats or unsaturated fats. Foods like butter, coconut oil, and animal fats are saturated fats. Saturated fat isn't bad. You actually need some, but it's inserted into a lot of food already, so the challenge is to start incorporating the unsaturated fat in order to balance things out a bit.

Which nuts/cheeses/dressings do I like to eat?

I personally love almonds, cashews, and peanuts. Walnuts and any nut is perfectly fine to eat. The more natural, the better though. Prepackaged trail mixes tend to have a lot of salt and sugar already added, so it's best to buy your nuts as raw as you can get and mix them yourself for your own trail mix.

Cheeses and dairy products are okay. Depending on your body type, you may be able to eat more or less of this. Endomorphs can eat more. Ectomorphs should eat less, because they eat more carbohydrates and less fats. It doesn't mean you can't have it at all. You will find that the foods you should be choosing depend on your healthy balance for your body type and metabolism.

I am allergic to these foods:

When you are allergic to any food, I would recommend speaking to your allergist or doctor about your goals and what you would like to do. He/She will most likely have healthy options and ideas for you as to what you should eat instead. Thankfully, certain vitamins and minerals are found in all different types of foods, so if you are unable to eat a certain food, you may be able to get that nutrient in another. But it's definitely something you need to discuss with your doctor. Find out if you are deficient in any nutrient due to allergies and find a way to get what your body needs.

I get _____ hours sleep each night.

Sleep! The dreadful "S" word that we all wish we had more of, but don't seem to want to make it higher on the priority list. I'm guilty. I'm a night owl, and love to stay up, because night time is when my kids are fast asleep and I can drink my coffee and browse the internet in peace. But I also face the consequences when I need to get up early. I feel sleep deprived and cranky, which effects my mood and patience with my children and myself. I lose motivation, because I'm tired and end up talking myself out of workout out and caring less about what I put into my mouth. So does sleep have an impact on our health and fitness journey? YES! You need sleep. Sleep has a ton of other health benefits as well, but it does effect your progress. I recommend trying to get 7-8 hours of sleep each night. The more the better! Sleep is also where muscle recovery happens and your muscles rebuild and strengthen.

After reading through all my advice for each question, I hope you have figured out what it is that you are struggling with most. Know this...you are not alone. I didn't create these questions randomly. I have found that these questions contain the biggest obstacles but also the biggest solutions in our health and fitness journey. If we can identify our own issue, then we can actively start working on that obstacle and develop a strong healthy foundation. You can do this!

Below, I will be giving you the opportunity to put this advice to action. That's what it takes. You may know what you need to work on, but are you willing to WORK! I hope the answer is yes, because you are worth it. You deserve this! It is NOT Impossible! It just takes one day at a time and a conscious effort to try!

<u>21 Day Challenge to Building Healthier Habits:</u>
<u>Biggest Obstacle</u>

My WHY:

_____

My GOAL:

_____

My OBSTACLE (PICK ONLY ONE) that I want to make healthier:

_____

START DATE: _____   END DATE: _____

Check off the box when you complete each day. Next to the day, write what you did to improve your unhealthy habit. It could be anything from choosing a healthier option to choosing not to have that food/drink at all. Write down what you did. Be intentional and specific with your answers. Honesty and commitment is what will help you truly transform your habits.

☐ Day 1:

_____

☐ Day 2:

_____

☐ Day 3:

_____

☐ Day 4:

_____

☐ Day 5:

_____

☐ Day 6:

_____

☐ Day 7:

_____

You have completed a week of improving your habits! You are awesome! Reflect a bit and figure out what you can improve even more!

What were some of the thoughts that kept creeping into mind during this process? If this is easy for you, then you're not working hard enough. It's a challenge for a reason. Great things happen when we push outside of our comfort zones. Get uncomfortable, attack this obstacle, and keep on trying! You can do it!

Bring on the next 7 days!!! YOU GOT THIS!

☐ Day 8:

_____

☐ Day 9:

_____

☐ Day 10:

_____

☐ Day 11:

_____

☐ Day 12:

_____

☐ Day 13:

_____

☐ Day 14:

_____

You've completed the next 7 days!!! Awesome job! Is it getting any easier? If you are struggling, have you found a healthier alternative yet? Are you encouraging yourself along the way? Or find yourself complaining. Mindset is key during your journey. Get that positive self talk back! Either way...Keep on going! You're doing great so far! You're pushing limits. You are testing yourself. You are forming new healthy habits. Don't Quit! Only 7 Days left in this Challenge!

☐ Day 15:

_____

☐ Day 16:

_____

☐ Day 17:

_____

☐ Day 18:

_____

☐ Day 19:

_____

☐ Day 20:

_____

☐ Day 21:

_____

WOOHOO!!! You have completed the 21 Day Challenge to Building Healthier Habits! You should be so proud of yourself!

How do you feel? Do you now have a good grasp on that obstacle? If not, don't be afraid to go through it again. We all run at different speeds. That's why YOU are in control. Don't feel bad about going at a slower pace. As long as you are genuinely working on it, you will start to feel a shift in your habits as they improve. If you do feel like you have overcame one of your big obstacles. I challenge you to do this again with your your next biggest obstacle. That's right. It takes time and work. But I believe in you and believe that, in time, you will replace all your unhealthy habits with healthy ones and build that strong healthy foundation that you need to discover a healthy you.

I am going to insert this challenge one more time for your second biggest habit. In my experience, I have learned that just by tweaking these obstacles, you can make great progress in your health and fitness journey. Take on your second obstacle, and see the magic happen. If you'd like, you can photo copy the pages of this challenge and use it as many times as you need for any obstacle you may have. Do whatever it takes to form healthier habits by overcoming these obstacles.

21 Day Challenge to Building Healthier Habits: Second Biggest Obstacle

My WHY:

_____

My GOAL:

_____

My OBSTACLE that I want to make healthier:

_____

START DATE: _____   END DATE: _____

Check off the box when you complete each day. Next to the day, write what you did to improve your unhealthy habit. It could be anything from choosing a healthier option to choosing not to have that food/drink at all. Write down what you did. Be intentional and specific with your answers. Honesty and commitment is what will help you truly transform your habits.

☐ Day 1:

_____

☐ Day 2:

_____

☐ Day 3:

_____

☐ Day 4:

_____

☐ Day 5:

_____

☐ Day 6:

_____

☐ Day 7:

_____

You have completed a week of improving your habits! You are awesome! Reflect a bit and figure out what you can improve even more!

What were some of the thoughts that kept creeping into mind during this process? If this is easy for you, then you're not working hard enough. It's a challenge for a reason. Great things happen when we push outside of our comfort zones. Get uncomfortable, attack this obstacle, and keep on trying! You can do it!

Bring on the next 7 days!!! YOU GOT THIS!

☐ Day 8:

_____

☐ Day 9:

_____

☐ Day 10:

_____

☐ Day 11:

_____

☐ Day 12:

_____

☐ Day 13:

_____

☐ Day 14:

_____

You've completed the next 7 days!!! Awesome job! Is it getting any easier? If you are struggling, have you found a healthier alternative yet? Are you encouraging yourself along the way? Or find yourself complaining. Mindset is key during your journey. Get that positive self talk back! Either way...Keep on going! You're doing great so far! You're pushing limits. You are testing yourself. You are forming new healthy habits. Don't Quit! Only 7 Days left in this Challenge!

☐ Day 15:

_____

☐ Day 16:

_____

☐ Day 17:

_____

☐ Day 18:

_____

☐ Day 19:

_____

☐ Day 20:

_____

☐ Day 21:

_____

WOOHOO!!! You have completed the 21 Day Challenge to Building Healthier Habits! You should be so proud of yourself!

Author's Note: I'd love to hear that you have completed the 21 Day Challenge to Building Healthier Habits and how it has effected you. I'd love to hear what obstacle you overcame and what your healthier option is. I'd love to be able to congratulate you personally and offer any other tips and tricks related to your obstacles as well. Feel free to e-mail me so we can celebrate together! katy.katydidfitness@gmail.com

Chapter 13

YOUR CALORIC INTAKE

It's supposed to be hard. If it wasn't hard, everyone
would do it. The hard...is what makes it great."
-A League Of Their Own

Up until this point, we have discussed basic daily
habits of improving your health and worked on
actually improving those habits. Now, we will take
that one step further and you will learn more about
your own caloric intake and how to adjust it according
to your personal health and fitness goals.

Did you know that your body burns calories while
you're resting? Sure, your body burns calories at a lot
slower rate, but it still burns calories while you sleep.
Your body burns calories at a faster rate as you move
and exercise. That is why exercise is important in
weight-loss goals.

Weight-loss is based on a calorie-in, calorie-out
philosophy. If you burn more calories than you eat,
then you will lose weight. If you eat more calories
than you burn, you will gain weight. And if you burn
the same number of calories than you eat, then you

will maintain your weight.

You may not like to track the output and input of calories. More often than not, I find my clients are actually eating way less than their body needs, putting their body in starvation mode. Not surprising, this is very common since the idea of eating is associated with weight gain, and individuals are afraid that if they eat, then they will gain weight, which is just not true. If your body enters starvation mode from under-eating, then your body stores that food as fat, because your body doesn't know when it will get food again. Your body is trying to conserve that energy for survival.

Activity level also depends on how many calories you can consume. Below is a formula that will help you figure out an appropriate calorie range for your daily activity level and fitness goal.

Calculate Your Calorie Range:

	Goal: Weight-loss	Goal: Maintain	Goal: Gain Weight
Sedentary (minimal exercise)	Body weight (lb) x 10-12	Body weight (lb) x 12-14	Body weight (lb) x 16-18
Moderately Active (3-4 times/wk)	Body weight (lb) x 12-14	Body weight (lb) x 14-16	Body weight (lb) x 18-20
Very Active (5-7 times/wk)	Body weight (lb) x 14-16	Body weight (lb) x 16-18	Body weight (lb) x 20-22

Example: A 156 lb woman who is currently sedentary and wants to lose weight will insert her weight into the formula: body weight (156 lb) x 10 = 1560 and do it again in with the higher number. 156 x 12 = 1872.

This woman's daily caloric intake range is 1560-1872 in order to start losing weight.

Let's Take Action:
It's time for you to figure out your daily caloric intake range. This will give you a basis as to where to start with narrowing down and targeting your specific goals.

Current Body Weight: _____ lbs

Goal (circle one):
Weight-loss, Maintain Weight, Gain Weight

Activity Level (circle one):
Sedentary, Moderately Active, Very Active

Use the formula from the chart above to calculate your caloric range:

_____ lb x (lower number in range)_____ = _____

_____ lb x (higher number in range)_____ = _____

Your Caloric Range is between: _____ and _____

This is simply your starting point. As you move closer towards your goal, you will want to recalculate the numbers. I would recommend doing this at the beginning of each month.

Now that you have figured out your personal daily caloric intake range that you should be eating, how are you going to track this? You can look at the nutrition labels and write them down on a piece of paper as you eat throughout the day. You can also use a nutrition app to track your food. Most nutrition apps at least have the calorie tracker where it keeps track of your calories for you.

You have already started developing healthier habits with your daily meals by overcoming your big obstacles from the previous chapter. However, making sure your caloric intake is in line with your goals is a very important aspect to a healthy nutrition as well. Simply calculating how many calories you eat in a day will help you become more aware of the calories in different foods and help you make better choices. If you pick foods with less calories, you can eat more of it. If you pick higher calorie foods, you will find yourself hungry by the end of the day, because once you hit your calorie limit you should stop for the day and only drink water.

Remember this is the basic principle of calorie counting. This is not where your journey with nutrition should end. It is simply one of the stepping stones that you can work on and create routine before you're ready to get more complex.

Not all low calorie foods are created equal. Just because you select a low calorie option, doesn't mean that it has the nutrients your body needs. It could just be full of empty calories to get you through a day, but provide no nutritional value what so ever. 100 calorie dessert snack packs and rice cakes are a great example of this. So keep this in mind as you begin to start counting calories. Start off staying within the calorie range, then work your way into asking yourself if this food that you are choosing contains helpful nutrients for your body. That little question will help you start making better choices as well.

Let's Take Action:

For the next 3 days, I challenge you to calculate the calories you eat. Read the labels and write down the calories for each meal/food/drink that enters your mouth. Fill in the chart below to see if you are within your targeted caloric range.

My Caloric Range: _____

Day 1:

	Record of Calories for foods tracked	Total Calories per Meal
Breakfast		
Snack		
Lunch		
Snack		
Dinner		
Snack		
		TOTAL:

Total Calories For Day 1: _____

Am I Within My Range: YES   NO

How many calories am I over or under?

My Caloric Range: _____

Day 2:

	Record of Calories for foods tracked	Total Calories per Meal
Breakfast		
Snack		
Lunch		
Snack		
Dinner		
Snack		
		TOTAL:

Total Calories For Day 2: _____

Am I Within My Range: YES   NO

How many calories am I over or under?

My Caloric Range: _____

Day 3:

	Record of Calories for foods tracked	Total Calories per Meal
Breakfast		
Snack		
Lunch		
Snack		
Dinner		
Snack		
		TOTAL:

Total Calories For Day 3: _____

Am I Within My Range: YES   NO

How many calories am I over or under?

Calorie counting is slightly more complex than building basic healthy habits, but it still only just a stepping stone to the greater picture of a healthy you. You started off by tweaking daily habits for the better. Then, you figured out the actual quantity of calories you should be eating according to your goals and tweaking your intake to make sure you are within that range. Next, you will make sure that those habits and calories are well rounded and filled with the macronutrients your specific body needs in order for you to accomplish your goals in a healthy and nutritionally balanced way. Are you ready?!

Chapter 14

YOUR MACRONUTRIENTS

"The food you eat can be either the safest and most powerful form of medicine, or the slowest form of poison." -Ann Wigmore

You're probably looking at this title and wondering what in the world are macronutrients. What diet is this? I promise you, this is not a fad diet. I used to think it was too. Guilty as charged, before becoming a certified trainer and really understanding the nitty gritty of nutrition. I spent a long long time tracking my calories. That's right. I stuck to the information from the previous chapter for years. That is actually how I lost all my baby weight after each pregnancy as well as all my other goals that I've done on my own. Counting calories. It totally worked, but I always seemed to find myself hungry by the end of each day and still had my crazy chocolate cravings. I wasn't sure why, or let's just say I thought I was supposed to be hungry at the end of the day. I mean...if I wasn't hungry, then I probably won't lose weight...right?

That mentality might get results, but it was all wrong. The sad part is, I never knew it until I learned for myself. I quickly learned that I was choosing all the wrong foods. I wasn't giving up the foods I loved. I still ate them whether they were healthy or not and just stopped eating after I hit my calorie number. We all talk about eating healthy and to have a balanced nutrition. But do we even really know what that means? That balance that everyone talks about actually comes down to the macronutrients in the foods we eat. But not everyone really means it that way. They just mean pick a healthy choice randomly throughout the day. No, a balanced nutrition is when the key macronutrients are set to a specific range for your body type and metabolism and you eat those macronutrients accordingly. That is when you will no longer have intense cravings and temptations. That is when you will find a balanced nutrition.

With that said, you're probably wondering what the heck macronutrients are and why are they so important. Macronutrients are the three main categories in which all food is broken down into in our bodies: Carbohydrates, Proteins, and Fats. Everything we eat falls into these categories. EVERYTHING!!! Our bodies need all of these to function properly.

Carbohydrates contribute to balancing our glucose level and is required for optimal performance.

175

Proteins help our strength, immune function, and weight management. Fats provide energy, balance hormones, and provide essential fatty acids that the body can't make on its own. Each micronutrient has an important role in the body, and without one of these categories, it would be hard to achieve the healthiest version of you that you are looking for.

This is why it is so important to have the correct balance of macronutrients in your body. From my experience, almost every woman that I've started working with has been extremely high in carbohydrates and extremely low in protein consumption.

Carbohydrates breakdown into sugar in the blood. Our blood can only store so much sugar. All the left over sugar finds somewhere else to go and is stored later...usually as the unwanted fat we have on our bodies. Protein is responsible for replenishing our amino acid pool that is constantly being drained, not only from workouts, but from everyday work as well. Our bodies do make some amino acids, but without the proper nutrition you may be missing out on 8 of the essential amino acids that must be brought into the body through nutrition.

With that said, your body performs best with a certain amount of each macronutrient. This is determined by your body type and metabolism. Earlier in the book you determined what body type you were: an ectomorph, mesomorph, or endomorph. Do you remember what you wrote down? If not, go back to Chapter 6 and look, because you'll need to know.

I Am This Body Type (circle the one you are)

Ectomorph   Mesomorph   Endomorph

Each body type breaks down and stores food differently, so it is important to make sure that you are eating according to your body type and what your body needs.

In the past, you may have been influenced by what your friends were doing to lose weight. Your friend may have lost 30 lbs cutting out carbs, but when you tried that method, you gained weight instead. Honestly, it wasn't until I learned about how macronutrients worked when I stopped caring what the world was doing and started focusing on what was best for me and my body. You may have a totally different body type than your friend. You may have a different activity level than your friend. These things make a difference!

I do want to make one thing clear: your body NEEDS ALL of these macronutrients! It is not a good idea to cut one out completely. Do you know what will happen? Your body will be deprived of it, you may become deficient in certain vitamins and minerals, and you will most likely start craving that macronutrient in the forms of bad foods.

I hear it all the time! I'll hear women say, "I'm doing this "so called" diet where I can't eat any carbs. I lost 20 lbs in 10 days!" Then, not that long after, they look over and see a chocolate cake! They fixate on what they can't have and it's pure torture. It's possible for them to stay strong for a week, but not sustainable long term and end up diving back into that chocolate cake like a kid in a candy store...indulging because they felt deprived and are sick of it...and gain back some of the weight they worked so hard to lose.

Don't do that to yourself. Why?! Your body needs carbohydrates to balance glucose levels, so rather than not eating it at all, try to find that balance that your body can handle.

Why is it that we always want what we cannot have? Do you feel that way? As soon as my husband hears the word diet, he is instantly hungry. As soon as the refrigerator looks a little bare, he panics and thinks we'll starve.

But imagine if you had a healthy balance of carbohydrates, proteins, and fats. Then you can still eat your carbs in moderation, you are no longer on a diet, but eating a healthy balance, and your body is getting what it needs to function properly.

I know, I know...easier said than done. And I'm sure healthy eating sounds just like a diet to you, but your body will not send signals telling you that you are hungry or deprived of something, unless you are. These signals may come as feeling nauseous, faint, headaches, hunger pains, cravings, and a lot of other not so fun side effects. Maybe not right away, but over time unhealthy eating will wear on your body in a negative way.

So let's find your healthy and break down the macronutrients!

There are apps to help you log your food and will do the calculations for you. A lot of apps provide a general breakdown for your height and weight...you'll notice they don't ask you for your body type. Those can be misleading at times. In general, they will work, but if you can get more specific to your body type and metabolism, that's even better.

Depending on what body type you are, you will get a percentage breakdown for each category. This will help you get an idea of what your portion sizes should look like. I recommend using your hands as a guide for portion control. Why? Well, your hand is proportionate to your body. Bigger people need more food. Smaller people need less food. Also, your hands go with you everywhere. You cannot make excuses saying that you left your portion containers at home.

I will provide a food list at the end of this chapter to help you make healthy choices for each category. You will be able to write in the portion that is appropriate for you in each category.

Ectomorphs: You should have your allotted calories from the previous chapter to reach your weight goal. Your macronutrients should be: 55% carbohydrates, 25% protein, and 20% fat. If you are an ectomorph, then you need more carbohydrates than fats. That is something to note. Your portions should be 1 palm of protein dense foods, 1 fist of vegetables, 2 cupped handfuls of carbohydrate dense foods, and a 1/2 thumb of fat dense foods.

Mesomorphs: You should have your allotted calories from the previous chapter in order to reach your weight goal. Your macronutrients should be: 40% carbohydrates, 30% protein, and 30% fat. If you are a mesomorph, then your portions should be pretty even. Your portions should be 1 palm of protein dense foods, 1 fist of vegetables, 1 cupped handful of carbohydrate dense foods, and 1 thumb of fat dense foods.

Endomorphs: You should have your allotted Calories from the previous chapter to reach your weight goal. Your macronutrients should be: 25% carbohydrates, 35% protein, and 40% fat. If you are an endomorph, then you need more fat-dense foods than carbohydrates. That is something to note. Your portions should be 1 palm of protein dense food, 1 fist of vegetables, a 1/2 cupped handful of carbohydrate dense foods, and 2 thumbs of fat dense foods.

Working on a balanced nutrition for your specific body type will keep you moving towards your goal in a healthy way.

Previously, I had mentioned metabolism along with body type when determining which breakdown you should follow. If you are over the age of 30 and you have a sedentary lifestyle then your metabolism is slower than it used to be and I would recommend you start with the endomorph breakdown.

It doesn't matter what your body type is if you have been sedentary for a long time. Your metabolism has learned to slow down to coincide with your energy burn, which isn't a lot. This means that you would not burn carbohydrates very well because carbohydrates are a slow burning energy. That is why runners need more carbohydrates, because the carbohydrates stay in their system longer and gives the energy they need for long endurance runs. But an individual who is sedentary or does very little cardio or exercise would not burn off the carbs fast enough and would most likely store it as fat.

An endomorphic breakdown allows for a higher healthy fats percentage. Healthy fats are fast burning energy, so the body will be able to get energy from healthy fats but burn and use them in an individual who has a slower metabolism, so it doesn't store in the body as fat deposits. No matter what you ate when you were younger and could get away with eating, a slower metabolism and inactive lifestyle won't allow you to eat the same way you used to eat as a kid.

It's Time To Take Action: Answer the questions honestly in order to pinpoint where you can improve.

Which category do I eat more than others? (circle one)
carbohydrates   proteins   fats

My macronutrient breakdown should be:

____ % carbohydrate _____% protein _____% fat

My calorie range should be _____.

Now enter your high caloric number into the formula in order to calculate your high grams. And enter your low caloric number to get your low grams.

High Calories ✖ % of carbs= _____ ÷ 4 = grams of carbs

Low Calories ✖ % of carbs= _____ ÷ 4 = grams of carbs

High Calories ✖ % of protein= _____ ÷ 4 = grams of protein

Low Calories ✖ % of protein= _____ ÷ 4 = grams of protein

High Calories ✖ % of fats= _____ ÷ 9 = grams of fats

Low Calories ✖ % of fats= _____ ÷ 9 = grams of fats

Example:

1800 ✖ .25= 450 ÷ 4= 122.5g of carbs

1550 ✖ .25= 387.5 ÷ 4= 96.8g of carbs

Carbohydrate Range = 97g-123g

1800 ✖ .35= 630 ÷ 4= 157.5g of protein

1550 ✖ .35= 542.5 ÷ 4= 135.6g of protein

Protein Range= 136g-158g

1800 ✖ .40= 720 ÷ 9 = 80g of fat

1550 ✖ .40= 620 ÷ 9= 68.8g of fat

Fat Range= 69g-80g

Here are some ways to help you track your food:

1. Only track calories. Write the calories while you eat and stop when you hit your allotted number.

2. Only track macronutrients. Write down the grams of macronutrients while you eat and stop when you hit your allotted number.

3. Use appropriate hand portions to manage your portion sizes better.

4. Utilize a mobile app to track your calories and macronutrients with an easy visual to help you reach your daily goal of balanced nutrition.

Next are healthy food ideas. Write in the portions that fit your body type. Please note that carbohydrates include vegetables and fruits. If you find yourself eating only from those categories, make sure to incorporate more proteins and healthy fats into your nutrition.

Each meal in my day (eating 4 meals) **should consist of:**
_____ palm of protein dense food
_____ fist of vegetables
_____cupped handle of carb dense food (starchy carbs or fruits)

_____ thumb of fat dense foods

Fill in the Portions and Circle the foods in the list that you would eat. Then add the food you circled onto your grocery list!

Carbohydrates	Proteins	Vegetables
Portion-	Portion-	Portion-
___ cupped handful	___ palm	___ fist size

Carbohydrates

- Sweet Potatoes
- Yams
- Quinoa
- Couscous
- Kidney Beans
- Black Beans
- Lima Beans
- White Beans
- Lentils
- Refried beans
- wild rice
- Red Potatoes
- Mashed potato
- Corn
- Buckwheat
- Barley
- Oatmeal

WHOLE GRAIN FOODS
- Tortilla
- Bagel
- English Muffin
- Pancakes
- Waffles
- Pita Bread
- Bread
- Cereal
- Crackers
- Pasta

Proteins

- Skinless Chicken Breasts
- Turkey Breast
- Duck Breast
- Lean Ground Chicken
- Lean Ground Turkey
- Catfish
- Tilapia
- Halibut
- Cod
- Salmon
- Mahi Mahi
- Eggs 1 whole
- Egg Whites
- Greek Yogurt
- Yogurt
- Shrimp
- Crab
- Lobster
- Clams
- 95% Lean Ground Beef
- Tofu
- Pork Tenderloin
- Tuna in water
- Ricotta cheese
- Cottage Cheese
- Protein Powder
- Veggie Burger
- Turkey Bacon

Vegetables

- Pico De Gallo
- Brussel Sprouts
- Mushrooms
- Lettuce
- Celery
- Cucumbers
- Cabbage
- Okra
- Eggplant
- Artichokes
- Cauliflower
- Carrots
- Banana Peppers
- Peppers
- Green Beans
- Squash
- Tomatoes
- Asparagus
- Broccoli
- Spinach
- Collard Greens
- Kale

Fats	Fruits	FREE FOODS
Portion-	Portion-	Portion-
____ thumbs	____ cupped handful	unlimited

Fats	Fruits	FREE FOODS
- Avocado	- Applesauce	- Water
- 12 Almonds	- Pumpkin	- Lemon Juice
- 8 cashews	- Honeydew Melon	- Lime Juice
- 14 whole peanuts	- Figs	- Vinegars
- 20 pistachios	- Papaya	- Mustard
- 4 walnuts	- Banana	- Parsley
- Hummus	- Pineapple	- Cilantro
- Coconut milk	- Pears	- Spices
- Feta Cheese	- Nectarine	- Garlic
- Goat Cheese	- Plum	- Ginger
- Cheddar	- Peach	- Green Onion
- Provolone	- Mango	- Jalapeños
- Monterey Jack Cheese	- Kiwi	- Hot Sauce
- Parmesan	- Grapes	- Flavor Extracts
- Pumpkin Seeds	- Cherries	- Mrs. Dash Seasonings
- Sunflower sends	- Grapefruit	
- Sesame Seeds	- Apricots	
- Flaxseed	- Apple	
- Chai Seed	- Tangerine	
- Pinenuts	- orange	
- Olive oil	- Cantaloupe	
- Coconut oil	- Watermelon	
- Flaxseed oil	- Pomegranate	
- Walnut oil	- Strawberries	
- Pumpkin seed oil	- Blackberries	
- Peanut Butter	- Blueberries	
- Almond Butter	- Raspberries	
- Butter		
- Mayo		

You have officially created your own healthy grocery list! That is amazing! When you master this chapter, you will be unstoppable with your goals! It will take time and adjustments along the way. Remember that I was counting calories for many years before I started taking on the Macro balance and staying consistent long term. Be patient with yourself. Move at your own pace and take on a task you think you're ready for. Every step you take in this book will guide you one step closer to the healthy you are trying to achieve.

Chapter 15

YOUR SUPPLEMENTATION

"Nearly all disease can be traced to a nutritional deficiency." -Dr. Linus Pauling

When starting down the "diet" path, many assume that pills and powders are an automatic extra that needs to be incorporated into your life in addition to healthy eating. However, this is not the case. With a healthy balance in your nutrition and incorporating more nutrient dense foods, you will be automatically adding vitamins and minerals to your daily diet without even realizing it.

Unfortunately, with the hustle and bustle of life, the temptation and ease by which you can make unhealthy choices that lack nutrients just to get us through the day, result in vitamin and mineral deficiencies. These deficiencies will result in supplementations involving pills and powder. The key is to find out what you may be deficient in and eat foods that contain that vitamin or mineral. For example, if you are deficient in calcium, you can get that mineral through green vegetables, soybeans, nuts/seeds, fish, and dairy. There is a food out there with the vitamin or mineral that you may need. After trying to increase your levels for that deficiency with real food, your doctor may then recommend whether you may need to supplement depending on some test results.

You are different than everyone else, so you may need different things, but there are a few different supplements that are generally good for everyone to incorporate.

The first supplement is protein. Yes, it does come in a powder, but let me explain why this is an important supplementation. This supplement is recommended because the amount of protein that an individual needs is .8g per pound of body weight. I weigh 123 lbs. That means I would need to eat about 98g of protein every day. That is extremely difficult to do by solely eating nutrient dense proteins each and every day, while living an always on the go lifestyle.

Incorporating one protein shake a day allows you to reach your recommended number more easily. Now, there are a huge variety of protein powders out there depending on whether you are vegan or not, or prefer whey or soy. It's up to you which kind you'd like to use or prefer. I look for a protein that has at least 24g of protein in one scoop. Once again, you eat differently than me, so it is important to figure out how many grams would benefit you.   Also, if you are going through menopause, you might want to try a soy protein to help balance your estrogen needs.

Fish oil is rich in DHA and EPA, which are two omega-3 fats that help decrease inflammation, increase your metabolic rate, improve fat burning, increase carbohydrate storage in the muscle, and even help manage back and neck pain, among many other benefits. It is definitely beneficial to incorporate this into your nutrition.

Multi-vitamin and multi-mineral supplements are helpful to cover a broad spectrum of vitamins and minerals. This is not to treat a specific deficiency or cure a disease. This is a well-balanced supplement that provides you with multiple vitamins and minerals that your body needs.

A Greens Supplement helps with those who can't seem to eat their veggies. Veggies play an important part in getting vitamins and minerals, so if you are not getting those in your daily veggies, then a supplement may be necessary.

It's Time To Reflect: Think about your daily eating habits.

I eat more fresh foods or packaged foods?

If you chose fresh foods, then you're on the right track and you may want to adjust your portion sizes or expand your variety of choices to incorporate more nutrients into meals.

If you chose packaged foods, then I suggest that you start shopping around the perimeter of the grocery store. That is where you will find the fresh and frozen produce. Fresh is best, but if it's too expensive or it goes bad too quickly in your house, then frozen is the next best choice.

Do I eat protein with every meal?

If yes, then you may be getting enough grams of protein into your diet.

If not, then a protein supplement of your choice would be highly recommended.

I still have a protein shake as a snack even though I really try to eat meat with every meal. Not all meats are created equal. If you eat lunch meats, while on the run, then you may not be getting enough grams of protein.

I know I am deficient in these vitamins and minerals:

If you don't know, I would definitely take a multi-vitamin to cover all the bases.

If you are having some health issues and concerns, then check with your doctor to see what you may be deficient in. That will give you insight on what foods you may be able to start incorporating into your diet.

Chapter 16

THE POWER LIES IN YOU

"If you do what you've always done, you'll get what you've always gotten." -Anthony Robbins

This is it! You have been given the tools to help you succeed in your journey, but the power lies in you. It is up to you to put these ideas into action. I have given you the basic foundation in creating healthy habits, but ultimately it is you that will take you there!

If you have taken this book seriously and have honestly completed each reflecting section and challenge, then you are on your way to reaching your goals.

I will let you in on a secret. This isn't easy. You cannot just go through this book one time and expect to reach your goal by the end. These are tools to help you keep going. Practice incorporating these ideas until you find a way that works for you and they have become routine. Work on a section until it feels easy, because if it feels like a chore, then it's not a habit yet. Keep working on it. When your journey starts getting tough, go back and work on your mindset and positive self-talk, because ultimately it is your mindset that will talk you into continuing or allow you to get off track. There is a quote that speaks true to my heart. "You cannot fail, unless you quit." -Abraham Lincoln. No one is perfect. No one gets it right the first time. You practice and tweak until you get it right and it feels good. Remember your WHY and your goal and keep on trying!

Before you know it, the magic will happen.

*You will look less and less at your calendar, because your workouts will fit more naturally into your daily routine.

*You will have to track your food less and less because you generally eat the same things every day and you have learned the difference between healthy and unhealthy choices.

*You will be stronger, because you will be exercising with purpose and according to your goal.

*You will have the energy you were looking for.

*You will start celebrating your successes and your journey with others.

That my friend, is the foundation for the healthy you that you've been looking for. When you get to that point, you will have officially built a lifestyle of healthy habits and the power to have long term results.

Exercise Index

Ali Shuffle Punch
- Do alternating split jumps
- Punch forward with opposite arm to opposite leg
- Perform alternating movement quickly

Alternating Bicep Curls
- Place your feet shoulder width apart
- Keep your back in a neutral position
- Grab and hold the dumbbells with palms up
- Bend one elbow up
- Alternate between arms

Alternating Hammer Curls
- Place your feet shoulder width apart
- Keep your back in a neutral position
- Grab and hold two dumbbells
- Hold dumbbells like a hammer
- Keep upper body still
- Bend one elbow up
- Alternate between arms

Ankle Mobilization Seated
- Sit on a chair or bench
- Extend both legs
- Flex your toes towards your body
- Point your toes
- Repeat between flexing and pointing

Arnold Press
- Sit on a chair or bench
- Hold dumbbells with arms out at a 90 degree angle
- Press up into a shoulder press
- Bring elbows back to 90 degrees
- Rotate elbows to the front of your body while rotating palms towards your body
- Bring elbows back out to your side at 90 degrees and press up again with dumbbells

Ball Squat
- Place Exercise Ball Against the Wall
  Stand So the Exercise Ball is touching your lower back
- Stand with your feet shoulder width apart and slightly out in front of your body
- Lean back on the ball and squat into a sitting position
- Bend down until your knees are at a 90 degree angle
- Return to standing position
- Challenge yourself by holding dumbbells down at your sides

Ball Sumo Squat

- Place Exercise Ball Against the Wall
  Stand So the Exercise Ball is touching your lower back
- Stand with your feet outside shoulder width apart and slightly out in front of your body
- Point your toes slightly outwards
- Lean back on the ball and squat into a sitting position
- Squat down as far as you can go
- Return to standing position
- Challenge yourself by holding a single dumbbell in front of your chest

Bench Press with Dumbbells

- Grab and hold a dumbbell in each hand
- Lay on your back on a flat bench or floor
- Bend arms so your arms are at a 90 degree angle
- Extend your arms out over your chest

Bent Leg Core Rotation Lying

- Lay on your back on the floor
- Pull your knees up
- Place your arms on the floor
- Move your knees towards the ground to one side
- Bring your knees to back to center
- Rotate to the other side

Bent Over Rows
- Stand with your feet shoulder width apart.
- Bend at the hip at a 45 degree angle
- Hold dumbbells or barbell
- Bend elbows back, bringing dumbbells or barbell to stomach
- Squeeze back and keep back straight

Bent Over Toe Touch
- Stand up straight
- Bend your upper body at the waist to touch your toes
- Keep your legs straight
- Slowly return to a standing position

Bicep Stretch Standing
- Stand parallel to a wall
- Place the palm of your hand behind you and against the wall
- Extend your arm
- Hold this position

Bicycle Crunch
- Lay on your back on the floor
- Bring opposite leg to opposite elbow
- Alternate between two sides
- Exhale while you crunch

Bird Dog Alternating
- Position yourself on your hands and knees
- Lift opposite leg and opposite arm straight out
- Bring leg and arm back to position
- Lift the other side
- Repeat motion

Box Jumps
- Jump onto the platform
- Move your arms to assist in the jump
- Step off the platform

Bulgarian Squat
- Position a bench or stable knee level surface behind you
- Place one food back on the surface
- Position your front foot so you can squat down and not have your knee go over your toes
- Complete squat repetitions before switching sides

Burpee
- Stand up straight
- Squat down on the floor
- Assume the push up position
- Jump back to squat position
- Stand up straight

Butterfly
- Lay on your back on the flat bench
- Grab and hold the dumbbells
- Extend your arms straight above your chest
- Lower your arms out to the side
- Keep your elbows slightly bent
- Bring arms back to above your chest

Calf Raises
- Stand with your feet closer together
- Push up on the balls of your feet
- Come back down
- Repeat
- You can hold dumbbells or stand on a step to do these as well.

Chair Dips With Bend Legs
- Stand in front of a bench or a low stable surface
- Place palms on the edge of the surface
- Squat down while supporting your arms on the surface
- Situate knees at a 90 degree angle
- Bend your arms at a 90 degree angle down and back up

Chair Dips With Legs Elevated
- Stand in front of a bench or a low stable surface
- Place palms on the edge of the surface
- Squat down while supporting your arms on the surface
- Place your feet and mid calf on a bench or exercise ball
- Bend your arms at a 90 degree angle down and back up

Chest Stretch Standing
- Stand so one shoulder is against the wall
- Stretch your arm back so your palm and shoulder are on the wall
- Feel the stretch in your chest
- Switch sides

Close Push-Ups
- Assume the push up position
- Keep your back in a neutral position
- Place your hands inside shoulder width
- Keep your hands in a neutral position over your torso
- Bend your arms
- Keep elbows close to the sides of your body

Close Push-Ups On Knees
- Assume the push up position
- Keep knees on the floor while crossing your feet at the ankles
- Keep your back in a neutral position
- Place your hands inside shoulder width
- Keep your hands in a neutral position over your torso
- Bend your arms
- Keep elbows close to the sides of your body

Concentration Curls
- Sit on a chair or bench
- Keep your back straight
- Move your torso forward
- Grab and hold a dumbbell
- Place one elbow against the inside of your knee
- Bend that elbow
- Do one arm at a time

Cycling
- Riding a road bike or stationary bike

Decline Push-Up
- Assume the push up position
- Place both feet/toes up on a chair/bench/step
- Keep your back straight
- Do not arch your back
- Place your hands shoulder width apart
- Keep your hands in a neutral position
- Bend your arms

Double Crunch
- Lay on your back on the floor
- Bend your knees
- Place your hands behind your head
- Tighten the abdominal muscles
- Bring shoulders and feet off the floor
- Exhale as your crunch elbows towards knees
- Return parts to the floor before crunching up again

Dumbbell Calf Raises
- Stand with your feet shoulder width apart or slightly closer
- Make sure you can balance
- Hold dumbbells down at your side
- Slowly raise up on your toes
- Squeeze the calf
- Slowly come back down
- Try to keep your heels off the floor while completing your repetitions
- Use a step or lifted surface if you keep touching your heels to the floor

Eagle Supine
- Lie flat on the floor
- Place your arms on the floor out to the side
- Lift one leg straight up in the air
- Rotate that straight leg over the other leg so it is parallel to your opposite arm
- Bring your leg back to center
- Alternate between your legs

Floor Chest Stretch
- Get down on your hands and knees
- Place both hands far and wide in front of you
- Move your torso forward
- Feel your muscles stretching
- Gently pulse slightly up and down

Front Raise
- Place your feet shoulder width apart
- Keep nice and straight posture
- Grab and hold the dumbbells with a hammer grip
- Lift your arms forward one at a time
- Keep core tight to help with stabilization

Forward Bunny Hop
- Stand in front of the speed ladder (you don't need a speed ladder to do this exercise)
- Jump with both legs forwards inside the ladder

Heel To Toe
- Stand with your feet hips width apart
- Keep your upper body straight and stable
- Go back onto your heels
- Then shift to your toes
- Repeat while keeping stable

Hurdling
- Run forward
- Jump over the hurdles

Hyperextension Using Exercise Ball
- Position exercise ball on the floor close to a wall
- Position the exercise ball on your hips and lower abdominals
- Place your feet flat on the wall for extra support
- Position your hands behind your head or crossed in front of your chest
- Lift your upper body up off the ball and back down

Incline Push-Up
- Assume the push up position with your hands on a bench/stairs/table
- Keep your back straight and core tight
- Place your hands shoulder width apart
- Bend your arms

Jump Roping
- Stand with straight posture
- Grab the rope
- Rotate your wrist
- Jump up

Jumping Jacks
- Place your feet hip width apart
- Keep your arms next to your body
- Do jumping jacks
- Lift your arms sideways
- Spread your legs apart
- Move your arms and legs simultaneously
- Bring arms and legs back together simultaneously

Kneeling Thoracic Rotation
- Get down on your hands and knees
- Rotate your torso to one side
- Move one arm down, under, and across your body while you are rotating
- Pull your arm back and elbow up
- Repeat
- Do one side at a time. Do not alternate

Lateral In-In, Out-Out
- Stand in front of the speed ladder
- Step in and out of the ladder one leg at a time
- Practice increasing your speed

Lateral Raise
- Place your feet shoulder width apart
- Keep your back in a neutral position
- Grab and hold the dumbbells
- Keep your elbows slightly bent
- Lift your arms out to the side
- Focus on lifting from your shoulders and not your wrists
- Hands at shoulder height or slightly above to keep range of motion

Leg Extensions on Hands and Knees
- Position yourself on the floor on your hands and knees
- Keep back and neck in a neutral position
- Extend one leg back to a straight position
- Bend that leg in without touching the floor
- Extend out again until repetitions are complete
- Switch sides

Leg Swing Front and Back
- Stabilize yourself next to a wall
- Stand up straight
- Swing your outside leg back and forth
- Control your motion
- Turn and switch sides

Leg Swing Sideways
- Stabilize yourself next to a wall
- Stand up straight
- Swing your leg sideways
- Control your motion
- Switch legs

Lying Leg Abductors
- Lay on your side on the floor
- Keep your back in a neutral position
- Place one hand on the side of your head to prop yourself up a bit
- Place your legs in a slight pike position with your feet on top of each other
- Lift the top leg
- Control your motion
  Complete one side then switch sides

Lying Leg Adductors
- Lay on your side on the floor
- Keep your back in a neutral position
- Support your upper body on your elbow closest to the floor
- Lean back on your hip slightly
- Bend top leg so foot is flat on the floor
- Lift the lower leg so the inside of your food is to- wards the ceiling and your toes are flexed outward

Lying Leg Raises
- Lay on your back on the floor
- Extend both legs
- Place hands down at your side
- Keep your head in a neutral position
- Tighten the abdominal muscles
- Move your torso up and lift your legs
- Legs can either be bent or straight

Lying Toe Touch
- Lay on your back on the floor
- Lift your legs straight up with a slight bend at the knee
- Tighten the abdominal muscles
- Move your hands towards your feet and lift shoulders off the floor
- Touch your toes if you can
- Return torso back down to the floor

Marching In Place
- Keep your head in a neutral position
- Relax your shoulders
- Keep your back straight
- Keep your chest forward
- Walk in a relaxed fashion
- Lift knees as high as you can

Medicine Ball Chest Throw
- Grab the Medicine Ball
- Bring the medicine ball to your chest
- Extend your arms forward
- Let go of the medicine ball
- You can do this exercise lying down or standing while throwing it at an angled trampoline

Medicine Ball Hip Throw
- Grab the medicine ball
- Stand by a wall
- Place your feet in stride position
- Stretch your arms
- Rotate your torso towards the wall
- Rotate your feet along as well
- Let go of the medicine ball
- Catch the medicine ball
- Bring the medicine ball to your chest

Neck Stretch Sideways
- Keep your back in a neutral position
- Relax your shoulders
- Place one hand on the opposite side of your head
- Push your head to the side
- Feel your muscle(s) stretching
- Bring head back to center
- Stretch opposite side

Oblique Crunch
- Lay on your back on the floor
- Bend your knees
- Keep your arms straight down next to your body
- Lift your shoulders off the floor
- Move your torso from to the side
- Touching each hand to the outside of one ankle at a time
- Exhale contract your oblique muscles

One Legged Deadlift
- Grab and hold the dumbbells
- Stand up straight on one leg
- Move your torso forward
- Lift non standing leg back
- Keep your back in a neutral position
- Focus on balance and keeping your back straight with the leg that is rotating backwards
- Do one side at a time

Pilates
- Join a Pilates class at your gym

Plank
- Assume the push up position
- Drop down to your elbows while keeping a plank position
- Keep core strong and tight
- Do not let your lower back bow
- Position feet close or wide, whichever is comfortable
- Hold position

Push-Up
- Assume the push up position
- Place the hands at shoulder width
- Keep your head in a neutral position over your torso
- Bend your arms

Push-Up Clap Incline
- Assume the push up position on a wall or table
- Bend your arms
- Explosively push off the wall or table
- Clap your hands
- Land on your hands and bend arms for another push up

Push-Up On Knees
- Assume the push up position
- Place knees on floor
- Cross feet at ankles
- Keep your back in a neutral position
- Place your hands shoulder width apart
- Bend your arms

Reverse Crunch
- Lay on your back on the floor
- Keep your knees slightly bent
- Place your arms at your side on the floor
- Lift your buttocks off the floor
- Control the movement up and down

Reverse Fly
- Stand with your feet shoulder width apart
- Hold one dumbbell in each hand
- Bend over at the hips but keeping your back straight and abs tight
- Rest arms so dumbbells are touching each other in front of you
- Lift your arms sideways squeezing your upper back

Reverse Grip Bent Over Rows
• Stand with feet shoulder width apart
• Use dumbbells or straight bar
• Hold dumbbells or straight bar so palms are up
• Bend forward at the hips
• Keep core tight and back straight
• Pull elbows straight back so your hands touch your chest
• Return back to resting position

Rotating Lower Body
• Place one hand on opposite shoulder
• Place other hand on hip
• Move your hips from side to side while keeping your upper body straight

Running
• When in doubt always ask your instructor for advice
• Always request advice when starting a new activity

Russian Twist
• Sit on a mat or soft surface
• Bend your legs in front of you
• Lean your upper body back while creating a C shape in your back
• You will be sitting on your tail bone, so use extra padding if needed
• Hold hands together and in front of you
• Twist from side to side while keeping the rest of your body still
• Lift legs off floor for a challenge
• Hold a weighted plate or dumbbell for added resistance if needed

Seated Arm Shake
- Sit on a bench or chair
- Shake your arms
- Rotating your arms and hands towards your body and back out

Seated Double Bicep Curl
- Sit on a bench or chair
- Keep straight posture
- Tighten core
- Hold dumbbells with palms up
- Curl both arms up at the same time

Seated Double Hammer Curl
- Sit on a bench or chair
- Keep straight posture
- Tighten core
- Hold dumbbells with palms in towards body
- Curl both arms up at the same time keeping the hammer grip with the dumbbells

Seated Shoulder Press
- Sit on a bench or chair
- Keep straight posture
- Tighten core
- Hold dumbbells up at shoulders
- Press arms up over head and back down

Seated Tricep Extension
- Sit on bench/chair
- Grab one dumbbell with two hands
- Hold one end of the dumbbell securely behind head
- Extend your arms upwards over your head
- Keep your shoulders in fixed position
- Keep elbows close to your ears
- Bend your elbows
- Extend your elbows

Single Arm Tricep Stretch
- Stand with your legs shoulder width apart
- Lift one arm up and behind your head
- Gently press at that elbow with your other hand
- Fell a stretch in your tricep
- Switch sides

Single Leg Calf Raises
- Stand on one foot
- Use a wall for support if needed
- Rest the other food on the heel of the standing food
- Raise up on your toe and back down
- Try not to let your heel touch the ground

Single Leg Dynamic Stretch
- Lay on your back on the floor
- Tighten the abdominal muscles
- Extend both legs
- Bring one straight leg up towards your chest
- Grab your leg lightly
- Move that leg back down while the other leg comes up
- Alternate between legs

Spinning
- Ride a spin bike
- Participate in a spin class

Squat
- Place your feet at hip width
- Bend through your knees
- Keep your torso straight
- Keep your butt back
- Lift your arms forward and upwards
- Knees should not go past your toes

Squat Jumps
- Place your feet at hip width
- Bring your buttocks back
- Lower yourself until the upper leg is parallel to the floor
- Jump up
- Move your arms along

Standing Shoulder Press
- Place your feet at hip width
- Keep your back in a neutral position
- Grab and hold the dumbbells
- Place your hands outside shoulder width
- Palms facing forward
- Extend your arms upwards

Sumo Squat
- Stand with your feet outside shoulder width apart
- A wide stance
- Place arms on hips or in front of you to find your best balancing point
- Squat down
- Push with your heels when standing back up and thrust hips forward slightly
- Repeat

Superman
- Lay down on your stomach
- Keep your arms straight in front of you
- Place your palms on the floor
- Keep your back in a neutral position
- Tighten your lower back
- Lift your arms and legs at the same time
- Return to resting position

Swimming
- Choose a swimming stroke that is comfortable to you
- Swim from one end of the pool to the other
- Swim back and forth until goal lengths or allotted time is completed

Tricep Dip With Legs Extended
- Place your hands on a chair/bench
- Keep your legs straight
- Bend your arms
- Extend your elbow
- Keep your back in a neutral position

Tricep Kickbacks

• Stand with your feet apart
• Bend at the hips and support one hand on a chair/ bench
• Keep back straight
• Hold dumbbell in hammer position
• Rest arm at a 90 degree angle
• Straighten arm behind you while contracting your tricep
• Return arm back to 90 degree angle
• Complete repetitions for one side at a time

Tricep Stretch Behind Back

• Stand up straight
• Move your arms backward
• Weave your fingers together
• Stretch your arms

Tripling Heel To Butt

• Bounce in one spot
• Move one foot towards your buttocks like you are going to kick it
• Alternate feet quickly

Tripling High Knees

• Bounce in one spot
• Lift one knee up as high as you can
• Alternate knees quickly

Upright Row
- Stand with feet shoulder width apart
- Hold dumbbells/straight bar/ez bar down in front of you
- Hold the dumbbells/straight bar/ez bar with a narrow grip
- Keep your back straight
- Lift elbows up above shoulders while holding the weights
- Return slowly back down

W-Pump
- Place your hands in front of your belly button
- Keep your elbows bent 90 degrees and at your side
- Rotate your arms backwards to form a W shape with your arms
- Pull your shoulder blades together
- Bring hands back to your belly button

Walk On Balance Beam
- Stand on the balance beam
- Step forward one foot at a time

Walking
- Walk at a comfortable pace

Wide Push-Up
- Assume Push-up position
- Place hands outside shoulder width
- Keep back and head in neutral position
- Bend elbows

Windmill
- Place your feet at hip width
- Lift your arms out to the side
- Move your torso towards your one hip
- Rotate your torso to the side
- Alternate rotating from side to side

Yoga
- Join a yoga class or use the Katydid Fitness mobile app for yoga position ideas to create your own yoga workout.

Zumba Class
- Zumba is a popular way to get exercise while dancing. Join a class at your gym.

About The Author

* I am an ISSA Certified Fitness Trainer
* I am an ISSA Certified Specialist in Nutrition Coaching
* I am an ISSA Certified Transformation Specialist
* Published Author (find me on Amazon)
* I have a Bachelors Degree in Education
* I am a former 4 time INBA Natural Figure Competitor
* I am a busy Homeschooling Mommy of 3 kiddos

My dream is to incorporate my passion for teaching and fitness by combining the two and teaching women how to change their lifestyle and create healthy habits that help them reach their goals.

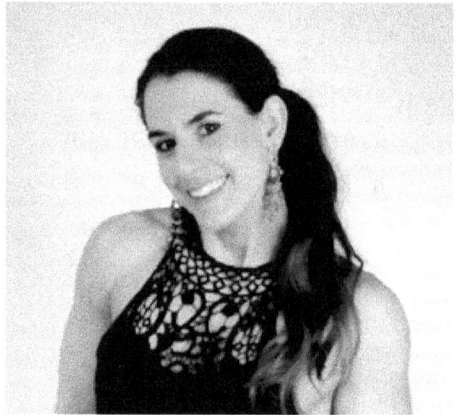

Let's be real! I've been working on my own health & fitness journey for over 13 years now. I've started from the bottom and worked my way to competitor status, bounced back after babies, and am now maintaining and working towards more specific goals.

I've learned through experience that there are different levels of exercise and nutrition and each level should be treated a certain way. It is my goal to provide you with resources at your level and teach you how to get to your goal, while maintaining a healthy lifestyle.

CONNECT WITH KATIE TEDDER

www.KatydidFitness.com

www.Facebook.com/katydidfitness

www.ingramcontent.com/pod-product-compliance
Lightning Source LLC
Chambersburg PA
CBHW062217270326
41930CB00009B/1771